WALKING

FOR FITNESS, PLEASURE AND HEALTH

WALKING

FOR FITNESS, PLEASURE AND HEALTH

A complete guide for women of all ages

HELEN VAUSE

FOREWORD BY DAME SUSAN DEVOY

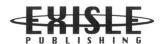
EXISLE
PUBLISHING

First published 2012

Exisle Publishing Limited,
P.O. Box 60-490, Titirangi, Auckland 0642, New Zealand.
'Moonrising', Narone Creek Road, Wollombi, NSW 2325, Australia.
www.exislepublishing.com

National Library of New Zealand Cataloguing-in-Publication Data

Vause, Helen.
Walking for fitness, pleasure and health : a complete guide for women of all ages / Helen Vause ; foreword by Susan Devoy.
Includes index.
ISBN 978-1-877437-13-7
1. Physical fitness for women. 2. Fitness walking. I. Title.
613.71082—dc 23

10 9 8 7 6 5 4 3 2 1

Cover and text design and production by Christabella Designs
Illustrations by Mark Roman
Printed in Singapore by KHL Print Co Pte Ltd
This book uses paper sourced under ISO 14001 guidelines from well-managed forests and other controlled sources.

CONTENTS

ACKNOWLEDGEMENTS

Many women with a passion for walking and wellness have made a contribution to this book by sharing their knowledge, networks and expertise. I would like to acknowledge them all for helping me to get started and for keeping me on track.

First, I want to thank Susan Devoy for her commitment and support and for welcoming me into the online community of Wonder Walkers with all of its great resources for walking women.

Early in the journey two of the Wonder Walkers experts in exercise, motivation, nutrition and so much more — Wendy Sweet and Christel Dunshea-Mooij — gave me generous attention and the vital professional input to help inform and shape the project.

I would also like to thank a number of women who have built businesses and careers out of being fit and well and have helped to motivate countless others to get active: fitness guru Michelle McCormack, Nordic walking exponent June Stevenson (Nordic Kiwi), Julie Renouf (physiotherapist), Jill Grant (A Walker's World) Carole Mills (Travel Managers), Jo Jukes (Oxfam), Yvette Higgins (Darebin City Council), Rachel Spriggins and Tanya Atkinson (Sport Wellington), Stephanie Moran (Vitality Works), Kirsten Andrews and Monique Blunden (Heart Foundation, Australia) and Sally Orr (London Moonwalk, Walk the Walk).

Without the assistance of these people, it would have taken a very long time for me to find the great bunch of women who patiently told me their stories (good bits and bad) to share with readers and hopefully to inspire others to become committed to regular walking and add another very healthy dimension to their lives.

Finally, a special thank you to Emma Darragh-Heath for allowing us to publish her lovely, poignant poem.

Helen Vause
February 2012

FOREWORD

The genesis of this book was the result of a website aptly named wonderwalkers.co.nz, which I developed with my colleague and friend Paula Thompson. I emphasise the word 'friend', because after all the trials and tribulations we have been through in developing this project, it is remarkable that we even talk to each other.

I moved to the winterless city of Tauranga in 2003 to take up a role as CEO of Sport Bay of Plenty. Sport BOP is one of about 16 regional sports trusts established throughout New Zealand to be regional arms of Sport and Recreation New Zealand (SPARC), the Crown entity charged with developing opportunities for people to participate in sport and recreational activities. The function of each regional trust is to be the local face of sport and physical activity. It was my first real job, apart from my earlier career as a professional athlete and my continuing role as a full-time mother of four boys.

Personal circumstances meant that suddenly my life was turned upside down and I was faced with the challenge of working full time, just when my youngest was about to start school. Instead of getting some time for myself, I was thrown head-first into the wonderful and complex world of management in the not-for-profit sector. It was both exciting and daunting: while the work was immensely rewarding, the sport and recreation sector was going through some major changes. And, as we all know, the not-for-profit sector is an enormously difficult environment at the best of times.

Not long after I had started my new job, Paula made an appointment to see me. She had previously been the CEO of Tauranga City Council and was now a consultant. I was sure she was looking for work, but I was impressed by her sincerity in welcoming me to town and offering her assistance if it was needed. 'Needed' proved an understatement: no sooner had I put my feet under the desk than I realised there was an overwhelming number of issues to deal with. I think I rang her the very next day. What followed was quite remarkable. Suddenly I was knee-deep in organisational restructures and hands-on learning about the principles of management, ably guided by one super-intelligent woman. In just a couple of years an organisation that could have shut its doors and no one would have noticed became a thriving and respected body, connected to its stakeholders and providing real added-value to the community.

Along the way our friendship developed, despite the fact our lives couldn't have been more different. But we did share a love of animals, particularly our dogs, and we felt most at ease when we were away from the office, out in the fresh air walking our four-legged friends. We soon found the walking meetings were far more productive than those held while fuelling ourselves up on coffee, and at every opportunity we would attempt to solve the problems of the world.

At that time we were mandated to encourage more people to be more active more often. The scope of our role was broad, from the couch potato to those actively involved in organised and structured sport. The then Labour Government was very keen to promote physical activity in an attempt to change our ever-increasing sedentary lifestyles and curb the onset of a likely obesity epidemic.

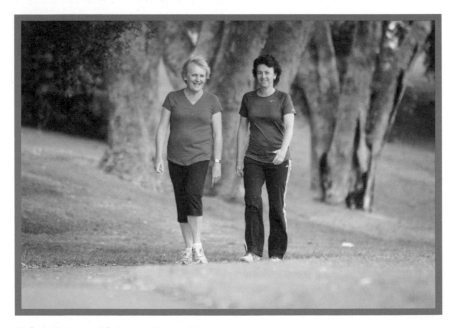

Helen Vause with Dame Susan Devoy.

Suddenly there were initiatives galore, and taxpayers' money was being spent indiscriminately on a whole raft of ideas aimed at improving our overall health outcomes. While we recognised the need, both Paula and I were doubtful about some of the ideas, and wondered if they were an indication of levels of bureaucracy gone mad. Was the message really getting through, or were people being put off by the unwelcome warning: 'Thou shalt exercise or thou wilt die'?

Unconvinced by the effectiveness of what we were doing, we knew our time at Sport BOP had come to an end. But rather than continue to whinge and moan about what we perceived wasn't working, we decided after many walks and many wines that we would put our money where our mouths were and take a giant leap of faith and have a crack ourselves.

So Wonder Walkers was conceived. Our over-arching goal was to find a way for women to enjoy being active, primarily through walking. Why walking? Because it is relatively easy, affordable, and good for the environment.

But at this time of my life there were personal experiences motivating me, too. I had become increasingly enthusiastic about walking, partly because of an accident that left me facing a long and arduous recovery and re-evaluating my options for staying fit and active. Even though I had long been retired from squash and the world of élite sport, I was still focused on being a super-duper athlete. I was out there running, challenging myself and looking for that adrenaline rush.

In 2007, all that went out the window overnight when I ruptured my Achilles tendon. Walking was very much part of my journey back to recovery. I really came to love it, by which time I had worked out that you don't have to go into oxygen debt and flog yourself in order to obtain great benefits from exercise. I also discovered that walking made me feel great.

I like to call walking my antidepressant of choice. But of course it's much more than that. It takes me into the glorious outdoors — a welcome change after years of exercising inside. It gives me time to think, it keeps me sane, and through it I have met many wonderful women who are walkers. And just like the rest of us, they all have their own stories.

When we set up Wonder Walkers we wanted it to be a place where women could get a daily fix of health without the guilt attached, and with a little humour thrown in. It is an opportunity for women to share whatever their hearts desire in a friendly environment. But we also wanted it to help plug that crucial gap that exists for most women between what we *know* is good for us and actually *doing* something that is good for us.

Over time we hoped that women themselves would become the queens of content and we would become a one-stop shop for everything to do with walking. Since the beginning, many wonderful women have contributed to Wonder Walkers. We have been overwhelmed by their humour and willingness to share in order to motivate others. And although we have a great group of experts in particular areas, the members themselves are also a formidable body of experts.

Frequently people have had experiences to share about walking that have been a really valuable contribution to the forum. And there is absolutely no doubt that many individual stories have set the ball rolling for others, who have just thought to themselves, 'Hey, if you can do it — so can I.' A success story from someone in one town has often prompted a woman somewhere else to take on a walking challenge. It's great to hear these tales from our members. And you don't need a string of letters after your name to make these things happen.

There are various reasons why women take to walking and to talking about it, but for many it is about their weight rather than the overall benefits. While we don't want to get fixated about weight loss, it's still pretty clear that many women put vanity before sanity. Yet so many still have very little understanding of the science involved in food, how their bodies work, and what their everyday eating has to do with that.

It is now widely accepted that obesity is becoming an increasingly serious problem and that there are thousands out there with undiagnosed Type 2 diabetes. It really isn't that difficult to develop the habit of healthy living and eating. Studies have shown the key success factors to be eating breakfast, walking, keeping a food diary and having support. That's the sort of formula we want women everywhere to understand.

Our goal is for walking to become the healthiest epidemic in town. It can be achieved, one step at a time. We learn as we go along, getting some wonderful feedback and being inspired by women who have made walking a part of their daily lives. We certainly want Wonder Walkers to contribute to giving women more understanding of how eating and moderate physical activity can improve their overall health status.

Wonder Walkers has been and continues to be a work in progress for me — in between four teenagers, a husband, a dog, not to mention washing, ironing, cooking, working and the myriad things any woman must do.

Like all good ideas, this project has inevitably given us some interesting learning experiences. Paula and I consider ourselves IT Luddites, and as time has gone on we have come to understand that with technology, the more you learn, the less you know. I freely admit that at times our enthusiasm has ebbed and flowed — along with our bank accounts, as we invested our own family silver, causing our fiscal Führer-partners to wonder if we had gone completely mad.

One thing is for certain: walking is finally being recognised as a valid form of exercise. It doesn't matter whether you walk the dog, whether you are a race walker or an avid tramper. When people ask if you exercise, you should no longer feel embarrassed to say you 'only walk'. More people these days walk in events than run.

The important thing is to do it regularly. We at Wonder Walkers believe walking is good for the body, the soul and the environment. It is a real winner.

Dame Susan Devoy, DNZM, CBE
Co-founder of Wonder Walkers
October 2011

Step by Step

Step by step
Troubles dissipate
Energy's restored
Words and fears and worries
Set free
Wafting away with the breeze of the day
Baby is sleeping — or quiet at least
Entranced by fresh air and nature's peace
Mother is moving
Step by step
Finding her rhythm, getting her groove back
A nice respite
In this new way of life
Along the track perspective appears
And what's that sound?
It's laughter I hear!
Loneliness fading
Music to my ears
For now, no cares
Just movement and mateship
and finding our way
Bit by bit Step by step Day by day
Everything's going to be OK
Walking is the way Walking is the way

Emma Darragh-Heath 2002

Chapter 1

INTRODUCTION

Walking has arrived well and truly as a very popular pursuit for exercise, health and fitness, for holidays and adventures. And it has taken on a competitive edge, too, among small groups of friends, individuals challenging themselves with pedometer readings, and the thousands now lining up to walk half-marathons and other events. It is no longer the default activity for women who are too unsporting or old to jog, cycle or hit balls, although it suits them well enough as an active lifestyle choice.

All over the world, where those out pounding pavements in the mornings and evenings would once have been mostly joggers, walkers are out there, too, in growing numbers. Governments and health organisations are reporting — and researching — big increases in the numbers of walkers of all ages, including those reaching midlife years and beyond.

Walking has a particular appeal to women for many reasons as they adapt to the changing stages of life — from pushing prams or combating work stresses, to battling their bulges and warding off ailments in later life. It suits women because it fits in throughout the balance of career and family, and because, more than most men, they like the social aspect of walking about in little groups, nattering, supporting each other and maintaining networks in this particular way. Whether you are the managing director of your own home and family, retired or in full career flight, walking is a great option for many women.

Smart, health-conscious women everywhere are working this out in their droves at all ages, but the baby boomers in particular are pulling on gear their mothers wouldn't have been seen dead in, to step out and keep up with life and wellbeing in every way. Walking is working for them because they can go as far as they like whenever they like, whenever they want and with whomever they like, to achieve all manner of goals. The motivation might be fitness, weight loss, companionship, better health, or a mix of all those things.

The surge in the popularity of walking didn't just happen overnight, although the really significant lift in numbers of walking women has come about in recent years. And like most things that become widely established in our lifestyles, the momentum has been kept up by a number of things that are all working together in the walking world and continue to recruit new members.

For example, walking has caught the attention of many researchers in universities who have run many trials on walkers of all ages. They are regularly reporting on the overall benefits of walking and enlightening us with more specific results on a whole variety of things from health impacts to social outcomes. Many governments and local authorities have got behind walkers, investing in the development of walkways and public health promotions to encourage citizens everywhere to embrace this trend in active living. Business has kept pace alongside in the sport and fitness sector, with a rise in sporting goods shops and products, personal trainers, sponsorships and special events. The media has been paying more attention to the subject too, and there are lots of websites and magazines providing useful, well-founded information to walkers everywhere.

In this book we take a look at the walking world, and talk to walkers and to some of the experts who advise them. Health benefits and walking techniques are obviously an important part of the story. Tips and warm-up techniques, well-designed step-by-step guides for building fitness and stamina, preventing injury and treating it when it does crop up, are points of interest, too. Many of the walkers we talked to had learned hard lessons about not paying sufficient attention to some of these things, and have either paid with injuries, failed to reach their goals or temporarily derailed their walking schedule. The walking wounded include the author of this book and getting back on my feet has invariably involved the support of a professional, or at least putting more thought into how I go and seeking relevant information.

Women who are serious about walking are interested in knowing more about how their bodies function. They are interested to know more about eating well and what foods to choose to sustain energy and to maintain a healthy body weight. For many, that includes getting good advice on how to lose the kilos that have crept on and kicked off the desire to get more active. And no book on walking would be complete without some tips and strategies from a motivation expert on how to get going and stay committed.

Walkers these days are less likely to be out in floppy track pants and any old sneakers. They are far better educated about the need to wear functional clothes and shoes, especially designed for their chosen activity. We consider the options, the good and bad choices in the bewilderingly large array of what is out there, and how to choose what's best for different conditions and individual needs. Before setting out with the credit card, wise women are looking up information on how to buy what will work best for them.

However the walking bug caught with women, a lot have been surprised at the effect it has had on their everyday lives, the fun they have had, the friends they have made and just how far it has taken them. A lot have stepped up the pace from a neighbourhood circuit to go further afield in groups or alone, to enter walking events or take wonderful walking holidays. Their walking, combined with the networks they have made and to some extent the ease of access to information on the internet, have propelled them much further than they had expected. Many a dream has been fuelled by reading the tales of others who have gone further, ahead of them, to reach big goals in faraway places.

We sought out many women at all ages and stages in life to talk about walking and its role in their lives. Not all of them feature in this book, and even though the stories they shared are about their own personal journey, they are similar to the stories of all women who walk and who have made similar discoveries on the way.

Our cross-section of women chose to start walking at different points in their lives, for a range of reasons that could be common enough to any of us. They wanted to get fitter and lose weight, and they wanted to get out with their babies and toddlers in the company of others like themselves. Some wanted to exercise and found groups and online walking buddies to jolly them along. For some, walking was the path to recovery from accident, illness or major life upsets. The going was tough, but the outcomes were rewarding for those who were working with serious health and weight issues.

They are an inspiring bunch of women who found motivation and determination. If they can do it, so can almost any woman with a body in reasonable working condition. We can all get walking if we want to, and we're likely to be very glad for years to come that we put on those walking shoes and made the decision to get going.

PROFILE

Turning life around with courage, walking poles and a pig-cell transplant

Karen Skinner found out she was an insulin-dependent diabetic when she was 24 years old. Over the next quarter-century she became a wife, a mother of three, a homestay host to international students, and worked at various part-time jobs. She ran a busy family and home, and had a big circle of friends, a regular exercise schedule, and an ongoing battle with her sometimes fragile and alarming health.

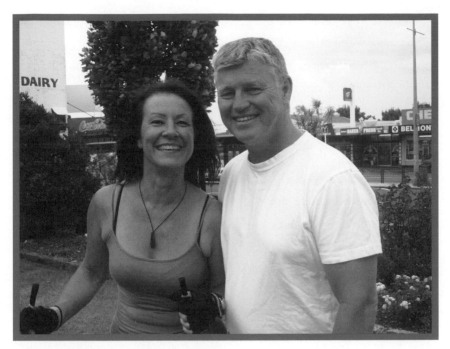

Karen and Ken Skinner out walking.

Approaching the milestone of her 50th birthday, Karen made some very significant choices in her search for options to potentially improve her health and wellbeing. In late September 2009 she was selected as one of the first four volunteers to take part in a controversial clinical trial that involved transplanting insulin-producing pig cells into her body as a treatment strategy for Type 1 diabetes. In June 2011 her journey through the pig-cell trial, and the very positive outcome it has brought for Karen, was the focus of the television documentary *Xeno*.

At the same time as she prepared for the clinical trial, Karen also decided to try Nordic walking in a bid to find an effective, fun and sustainable exercise routine that would be great for her health now and well into her mature years. It also needed to be a realistic exercise regime she could manage within her endless cycle of blood tests and the alarming swings in blood sugar levels that could suddenly plunge her into crisis, apparently without warning. Nordic walking would provide her with a good workout over a shorter time and distance than regular walking. Besides, her inability to sense the fall in her sugar levels made going out for longer periods downright dangerous.

Although very regular exercise and fitness had been a significant part of her very positive approach to living with diabetes — and battling the weight gain that comes with taking insulin — Karen had been pinning her hopes for some years on being selected for the pig cell trials. A year later, with the trial over, she's feeling fantastic and her dependence on insulin has fallen significantly.

The pig-cell transplant process was developed by Professor Bob Elliott at his research and development company, Living Cell Technologies. The expectation of pig-cell transplant is to greatly reduce dependency on insulin, or possibly even free people with Type 1 diabetes entirely from their daily regime of insulin injections.

The transplant process involved taking cells from the pancreas of piglets, coating them with seaweed gel and implanting them into the abdomen of patients, where they have been proven to manufacture insulin and help control blood sugar levels.

Professor Elliott's trial is absolutely pioneering stuff in research into the treatment of Type 1 diabetes, and the world of science (and diabetics) is watching with great hopes. The élite little group of piglets providing the cells for transplanting are kept in quarantine in the sub-Antarctic Auckland Islands, where the purity of the herd they are bred from has been ensured through about 200 years of isolation.

As number three of the first four selected for the trial, Karen was to start her year-long clinical trial on 19 January 2010, and the day couldn't come fast enough for her. Not surprisingly, this bright, positive and brave woman caught the eye of documentary makers and media keen to take her story and the controversial trial to the world. Quite often as they tracked her progress with the pig-cell treatment, the storytellers filmed Karen out and about on her Nordic walking poles, with her walking group.

Once the camera crew turned up, Karen had to fess up about her condition to her new walking buddies. 'I had always been very private about it, but at that stage I had to tell them and, although they had had no idea of what I was coping with on some days, they were great about it.'

Long before any thoughts of pig-cell transplants, Karen had kept up a walking routine in which all things — such as frequency, distance, fitness, level of commitment and walking companions — changed as her life changed apace with the growth of her young family. For a couple of years as a young mother, she had snatched time with girlfriends to stride along the beach on many mornings before daybreak. Whenever she lacked a walking buddy, she would set off for a few kilometres around the neighbouring streets, listening to her radio she went. In the evenings her husband, Ken, was a regular companion for pounding the pavements.

'I like to have company. Part of walking for me is socialising. Having a natter to women friends and catching up on our lives. And discussing things, too. I think that the companionship of walking with other women is an important part of the exercise to most women. Rather than facing silence or giving up and staying home, I'd have a talkback host along as my companion when I walked alone. But men can't be bothered talking when they walk. Ken says I'm always trying to get his attention about a hundred and one things because I'm so keen to talk to him on our walks,' laughs Karen. 'I know they think woman talk too much, but I just love the chance to chat as we go. It's all part of it for me. And, without a doubt, the enjoyment of company helps me to walk further and for longer periods.'

With the very big step of joining the pig-cell trial close to becoming a reality, Karen decided to check out one of the regular Nordic walking demonstrations held in the city by coach and advocate for the sport, June Stevenson.

'I wasn't quite sure why I had gone. It looked pretty strange, and at first I couldn't do it anyway. But I got the hang of it and then I loved it. This was going to be my new sport.'

Aware she would be wanting company out walking with her poles, Karen was quick to find a small group of others keen to master this style of walking and make a commitment to regular walks. Over a year later, they are meeting first thing on Saturday mornings at different locations for a vigorous walk — and of course a coffee and a catch-up. Often, they will walk for as long as three and a half hours, with the coffee stop already pin-pointed on their route. They try to go to new places and vary the terrain they walk on — flat paths, grassy parks, beaches and slopes, in whatever combination.

'We have all got much better at it, but you still have to think a little bit about what you are doing and how you are using your poles to get the most out of it. If you talk too much, you lose a bit of your technique.'

The benefits of the pig-cell transplant to date and the regular schedule of Nordic walking have combined to greatly improve Karen's overall wellbeing, her fitness, her strength and her figure. She estimates she's lost nearly four kilograms with the combined effects of the extra exercise Nordic walking gives over regular walking, and her drop in insulin intake.

'All round I just feel so much better. I feel very positive, I have more energy, I feel fitter, I have a clear head, and I am loving getting outdoors more often. The chance to be part of this trial has been fantastic, but the Nordic walking has been very much part of getting to where I am now at. Health is always front-of-mind for me: I never can take it for granted, and so I am always very keen to get out there and get walking.'

Chapter 2

WALKING FOR GOOD HEALTH ACROSS A LIFETIME

A raft of studies puts walking very high on the list of activities that boost our health and fitness and significantly reduce the risk of many health conditions. As we age it is also a proven and positive tool for battling whatever health conditions we might find ourselves facing.

For most people walking is a natural thing to do, and it is the natural way to keep our bodies trim, fit and functioning well, without the need for expensive gear or gym memberships. Trouble is, though, that we live in a fast-paced world where millions are bent over desks for long hours and whisk from A to B on four wheels. Getting about on foot is no longer part of daily life for many people — unless you count crossing the living room to the kitchen! Indeed, taking time out for a walk can almost seem to be a luxury. Yet walking is still essential to health and to living well. And, hectic lives or not, many are now realising it is an easy and practical way to keep organs working well and having a strong frame that is good for a lifetime!

Regular walking is a great habit at every age because it:
• improves fitness
• improves physical function
• strengthens the heart
• helps control cholesterol
• helps control blood pressure

- improves circulation
- helps keep bones healthy
- benefits the brain
- alleviates depression
- helps with stress management
- helps with weight control
- helps prevent disease.

While some health problems can arise in youth, the risks and the list of potential health issues get bigger as we move through the decades. Advocating and encouraging people to take up walking as part of an active lifestyle is a common theme in the health promotion messages of most leading health agencies and health foundations. These organisations make sure we are aware of the latest health research and the benefits of staying active, and some are leading the way by establishing walking groups for people of all ages and stages.

In Australia the Heart Foundation, for example, has invested considerable resources into setting up and promoting its very successful Walking for Heart groups right across the country. They now have about 1200 groups, and more than 16,000 lucky Australians are reaping the benefits of walking in groups that have been well organised and maintained for them. They report over 700 new members registering every month and an incredibly high retention rate of 97.5 per cent. They have set an enviable record and benchmark for other organisations in many countries who are working to get their citizens walking.

Therapeutic effects of walking

As well as having tremendous value in maintaining wellbeing and preventing or at least allaying some of the issues of aging, for millions of people walking is a recovery tool or support for coping with health problems. Following are just a sample.

Mental health

Walking releases those happy 'endorphins' that lift the spirits and help to relieve depression. It improves the all-round feeling of wellbeing, both physical and mentally. Walking in groups brings the added benefit of socialisation, helping to alleviate any sense of isolation. With a little practice, deep and rhythmic breathing also adds to the overall sense of wellbeing. Feeling better after a good walk is almost guaranteed.

Obesity

This is a significant issue across all age groups, and is the primary reason many a walker cites as their motivation for pounding the pavements. Many women battle all their lives with the balance between how much they eat and how much of it they burn off. Combined with a healthy diet, walking is an ally for many a woman in her personal weight-control programme. It is most effective when it involves brisk walking on a near-daily basis for at least half an hour.

Diabetes

Alongside the obesity bulge, Type 2 diabetes is on the increase in world health statistics. Regular walking is estimated to slow the risk of developing this condition by from 33 to 50 per cent.

Stroke

Most people who have strokes are into their senior years, and those whom it doesn't kill are often left with disability. While walking is an effective tool in recovery and regaining mobility, it is also been proven to help stave off the development of high blood pressure, which is a contributor to the risk of having a stroke.

Cancer

Walking and being active is shown to reduce the likelihood of developing a number of cancers, particularly bowel cancer. For many people who have had cancer, it has also been effective in lowering the risk of their disease recurring.

Osteoporosis

As women age beyond 50, there is a much increased risk of developing osteoporosis, which causes bones to weaken and break. Brisk walking with good posture is a great help to maintaining healthy joints and all-round strength.

Heart disease

This one is right up there with the most common causes of death. Regular walking helps keep the heart strong and helps in most recovery programmes from heart problems.

PROFILE

Breast Cancer Nordic walkers

In 2004, at the age of 41, Mary Anne found she had breast cancer. The cancer was beyond stage one, and she had a mastectomy but chose not to undergo chemotherapy. Soon afterwards she took a trip to Europe where she saw people out Nordic walking. It struck a chord with her, and she immediately wondered if this sport could be beneficial for women like herself. It looked like a great form of exercise for working towards rebuilding strength and increasing the odds against the likelihood of the cancer returning.

'We know regular exercise can be an important weapon in significantly cutting the odds of a recurrence of breast cancer. But Nordic walking has a particular benefit to women who have had mastectomies, because it engages the upper body and helps to rebuild strength. After a mastectomy you are left with scar tissue, and pain and difficulty with shoulder and arm function. Many find it pretty hard to use these parts, and try to protect themselves as they struggle with all the physical demands of daily life.

Yet it is vital to work on this to get back the full range of shoulder motion and get back into better shape.'

Mary Anne bought her poles in Europe and resolved to embark seriously on this course of self-help, but soon she realised she wanted to do more than go out and walk alone. She wanted to spread the word to other women in the same boat and get them out there walking with her. If she was to do that successfully, she would need to learn more about it first and be prepared to help others learn to use Nordic walking poles.

Back home she went to university and studied to become a personal trainer. She then set about establishing two now very successful Nordic walking groups for women who have had breast cancer and mastectomies. She had come up with the very sort of activity that had strong appeal, and a front-page photo and story in the local newspaper helped spread the word. Women battling other health issue were also welcomed into the walking group. Today there are around 40 members spread across two groups in her city.

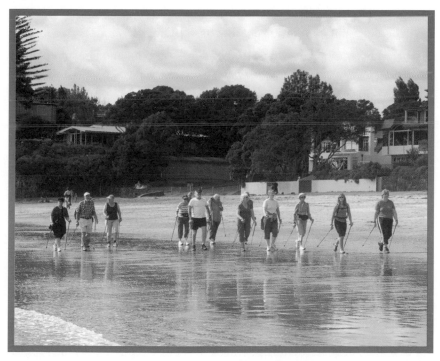

The breast cancer Nordic walkers walk along a beach.

They are a very determined bunch: rain, hail or shine, they are out there on the beach or nearby, doing enough laps to clock up at least 5 kilometres or more, and many do 8 kilometres. Both groups walk for an hour twice a week, and before and after they will run through a routine of warm-ups and stretches.

'Everyone is very committed,' says Mary Anne. 'No matter what the weather, we always walk unless our date falls on Christmas Day.'

Mary Anne provides the poles, because she feels first-timers might not yet be ready to make the commitment of buying their own, but she wants to give them every opportunity to take the plunge in their own time. She's a pioneer in this initiative and a volunteer, putting considerable time and work into her flourishing walking groups.

'I do it for love and because I can. I find it very rewarding to see women taking this up and getting stronger. Then they start to make bigger changes in their lives as they start to feel better or just plain start to feel great. Soon enough, plenty will be telling me that they are off to the gym, too, or that they have started doing pilates.'

'I call them the Nordic Talkers. Because of course women love to talk, and being able to do this when they need to — and feeling they are among friends who will listen and who understand — is a natural spin-off of our walks together. Often as not, though, it's not just cancer they are talking about; they just enjoying talking about all sorts of things, like everyone else. And being part of a walking group is a great way to keeping up motivation.'

One of her regular walkers credits Mary Anne with putting her on the path to better health and happiness. She says finding good company to walk with has brought her great enjoyment. It has also been a strong tool in managing her Type 1 diabetes and in her recovery from a mastectomy.

In the course of encouraging women with breast cancer to take up Nordic walking, Mary Anne has met others whom she realised could benefit from this sort of exercise if they were given encouragement and the opportunity. Recently she has provided that opportunity for a small group of women with brain injuries. Every week she takes a group of women walking who are struggling with recovering from the quite devastating aftermath of brain injury. For them the walking poles give them tools to get mobile, providing extra stability and overall support. While they work to improve overall fitness, they significantly increase the movement of muscle groups and the lateral mobility of the spine. They are an aid, too, to regaining co-ordination.

The eight women who have joined Mary Anne's group are aged in their 40s and 50s, and they are each tackling a range of post-injury issues on the tough road to recovery with her help and with the support of each other.

'We car pool to meet up in quiet flat places where they can try it in reasonable safety. We have to be very careful about the routes we choose, and we move pretty slowly, but it's very encouraging to see everyone trying hard and making progress. They would find it really hard to try doing something like this on their own. I just love doing this. I love to walk myself, but I get such a buzz out of working with all these women. It is a real privilege. Of course there are no guarantees for any of us, but trying is so much easier when everyone has support and a good plan for helping themselves.'

Chapter 3

MOTIVATION: FINDING IT AND KEEPING IT GOING

Happily enough, just reading about walking counts as doing something about getting started. So does sticking up on the fridge door an image of the trim, fitter woman who used to be you — or could be you.

Exercising the mind on matters of exercise without moving a muscle is an okay place to start on the first steps to regular walking. It counts in the quest for information, inspiration and motivation — things that lots of people take a while to find before taking up something new. And those yet to pull on their walking shoes will find plenty to read, written by both experts and ordinary folk, on mind games and motivation and exercise. There are strategies and tips aplenty out there, both online and on the book shelves, to get you on your journey.

Exercise psychology is a relatively new field, but it's a fast-growing area of both sports research and sports business. Wendy Sweet, a tireless advisor on the website for walking women, www.wonderwalkers.co.nz, is a recognised leader and educator in the fitness industry. With a master's degree in sport and leisure studies, and decades of experience in the fitness world, she is one of the new breed of highly skilled people who come up with the strategies to get people into long-term exercise.

Motivation is one of those things some people seem to have by the bucketful. But while some just need a shove to get going, for many people getting up the motivation to start exercising, and to stick with it, is all too difficult. They need all the help they can get from professionals like Wendy, and armies of others easily found in most towns and cities these days.

Gentle nudge or a powerful persuasion?

Twenty-one days is often quoted as the magic number for learning new habits, and this is widely considered to be close to the mark. It does not take long to learn new habits and make them part of your daily life, particularly if you are ready to, say the experts. But there is a big bunch of women out there who are much harder to get moving, even though they know it would be very good for them to get out walking. The experts have got this lot sussed, too. They know the excuses and can come up with heaps of suggestions to overcome the obstacles to exercise.

While the barriers might seem big, and some much bigger than others, where there's a will, there are a few quite practical ways to get around them. Sowing the seeds includes coming to an acceptance that you really do need to exercise, and understanding that doing it will really mean many good things for you. Positive thinking and a 'can do' approach will work wonders on these old chestnuts below!

Common excuses for not exercising

I'm overweight and I look awful

Making a start will obviously be the first step to dealing with this one. Getting nice gear to walk in will make you feel better about how you look. Find someone to walk with you in the evenings when you won't be so visible. Alternatively, walk very early in the morning. Consider driving somewhere out of your community where no one will recognise you. A hat and dark glasses could also help make you feel more invisible. You might make a wobbly beginning on this new journey, but once you start to feel benefits your confidence should lift. Remind yourself that you are walking yourself into a new woman.

It's boring

Walk with friends or an iPod, and vary the route or set off for an appealing destination, such as the shopping mall or a friend's house. Explore places you have never been to before. Text friends if you must, to amuse yourself as you go.

I don't have time

Most people with full and busy lives don't have a lot of time to fit in new things without making a real effort. Get up earlier, find a night-walking buddy. Walk at lunchtime or walk to work, and try walking on short trips where you would normally take the car. If you are tied to young children, take them with you and go buggy-walking.

I'm too tired at the end of the day

Just take a brief walk and see if it invigorates you. Walk at another time of day. Build up your stamina on holidays and weekends.

The weather is too hot or too cold for walking

Mall-walking is a great idea in very cold or very hot places where being outdoors is just too uncomfortable. If you are going outside into winter temperatures, dress well for the elements and chuck the walking gear in the clothes drier to warm it up a little before you set off. Warm up with a few minutes of exercises before you go out the front door. Beat intense summer heat by getting out first thing in the morning.

I haven't got anyone to walk with

Find someone. If friends are not keen or you are new to town, find a walking group. Get a dog for a faithful companion or walk someone else's. If you have to go it alone, listening to music or anything else you like could be all the company you need to make it much more enjoyable and interesting.

One step closer to those first steps

Whatever the barriers, many a new walker will have faced getting over one before becoming motivated and enthusiastic about their new routine and making it work for them. For the thousands who have made the commitment to get over themselves and their thinking around taking up exercise, most have made some change — large or small — to get going. Before they knew it, walking had become a part of their lives, with the benefits far outweighing any negative thinking.

Listen to the experts

According to Woody Allen '80 per cent of success is just showing up'. He has probably got a good point, but according to the health and fitness experts there are a few other things that can also help people become regular walkers and learn to love the habit.

Wendy Sweet says it's very important in the early approach to make a plan or a programme. The first three months are the critical period in changing behaviour, she says. After this, the new behaviour becomes embedded or forms a habit and the risk of relapse starts to diminish.

It is important, too, to have a goal and believe you can reach it. But Wendy also cautions that going at it too hard and too fast can end in tears for new walkers. And of course support is a big boost in tackling something new. Having your spouse, family, friends, workmates, teammates or maybe even a sponsor, to cheer you on is great for hanging on to motivation.

Get moving with these exercise motivation tips

Fitness expert Wendy Sweet offers the following advice:

1: Be realistic
One of the biggest reasons for failure is that first-time exercisers often set unrealistic goals. They want to go for big goals but tend to become overwhelmed. Do not start off trying for an hour every day. Instead, begin with 20–30 minutes of your chosen exercise two to three times a week.

2: Keep track of your progress
Don't forget to chart your progress, whether it is with a high-tech tracker or an old-fashioned fitness journal. Seeing incremental improvements — whether it's in improved time or greater frequency of workouts — can boost your exercise motivation. You can be inspired by seeing the value of what you do.

3: Don't expect perfection
Another pitfall is all-or-nothing thinking; a perfectionist's way of looking at life, which leads to giving up when you miss a day or two or when your workout doesn't go well. If you accept going in that there will be some sidesteps on your fitness journey, you will be mentally better prepared to deal with setbacks. Expect that you will get down from time to time, and be psychologically prepared to miss a few days of exercise when that happens. Do not let it be an excuse for giving up.

To keep injuries from sidelining you, do your best to prevent them by warming up, cooling down, and stretching properly — and not doing too much too soon.

4: Don't compare yourself to others

We have all seen them, those fatless specimens. Don't compare yourself or let them deter you from your goal.

5: Get support and find a walking buddy

It's about spouses, girlfriends, boyfriends and buddies — anyone who will encourage you. And if their encouragement goes beyond the 'atta-girl' approach, remind them you don't need nagging — just support.

6: Find the fun in it

It is essential to find an activity you like, and that doesn't mean sitting on the couch watching telly. Walking is the easiest exercise known to man (or woman).

7: Break it up

You can make it easier on yourself by splitting your exercise session into two or three sessions. Research supports the idea that this can be as beneficial as one long workout. So if you don't feel like going for an hour on any day, break it up into bits — every little bit helps.

8: Make it convenient

Do whatever you can to remove obstacles to exercise and make it as convenient as possible. Get outside for a quick walk when you can. Set your alarm a little earlier and walk in the mornings if you are too tired at the end of the day.

9: Forget the past

Don't let previous bad experiences with exercise hinder you. Maybe you weren't the most athletic person at school, but that was years ago. Your goal now is not to win a gold medal — you want to exercise to stay healthy and enjoy your life.

10: Reward yourself

Reward yourself for making the effort to exercise — not with a piece of chocolate cake, but with something you'll enjoy, perhaps a bunch of flowers or a movie. Try to think of treats which will reinforce a mind-body connection so you can savour the rewards of your hard work. Plan a shopping trip, or just an hour doing nothing. And remind yourself, with each precious moment, that you are enjoying this time because of all the great things you have been doing for yourself, and don't feel guilty about it. Of course there are lots more ways to keep your motivation up, whether it's rewarding yourself with a little retail therapy, dreaming of a fabulous new body by summer, the good feeling you get after exercise, or the discovery of blogging mates to talk about walking with. Not to mention stress relief, compliments from others, being able to squeeze back into favourite clothes. Or just the thrill of reaching your goals.

PROFILE

Lady Morrison: marathon-walking champion for Maori women's health

Fit, bold and highly motivated, 74-year-old Kuia, Lady Morrison has done many marathons since she first entered one in 1991 and inspired many others to take up the challenge with her. She has lost count of the walking events, but she certainly remembers why she does them and why she gathers up groups of Maori women to go with her on her walking adventures — be they modest or marathon-sized adventures.

'I do it for Maori women's health. I do it to help show the way to health and wellbeing for our women. I want to help turn around the negative statistics that currently apply to their health. Things like being too heavy or unfit or not motivated.'

And whether it is on the footpaths of her hometown Rotorua or the streets of New York, Lady Morrison has made walking her thing, a big part of her lifestyle and a motivator for many other women to make a commitment to exercise for their own wellbeing.

The Rotorua-based Morrisons have a long history as one of New Zealand's high-profile Maori families, and the late, legendary Sir Howard Morrison sang his way across decades of the country's entertainment history.

In her own way, his widow Kuia made herself heard, too, and just a month after Sir Howard's death, she managed to keep faith with her plans to lead a group of Maori women in the New York Marathon. Tough times aside, feeling ready or not, she showed up at the start line with her band of Maori women friends to walk her talk just as she had promised. It was no small ambition for Kuia, who was celebrating her 72nd birthday.

In October 2009 when she walked the New York Marathon she was an old hand at marathons, but with an older body, too. She felt the pain all right, but of course she made it across the line in typical style, tired but jubilant and up for adventures in the Big Apple.

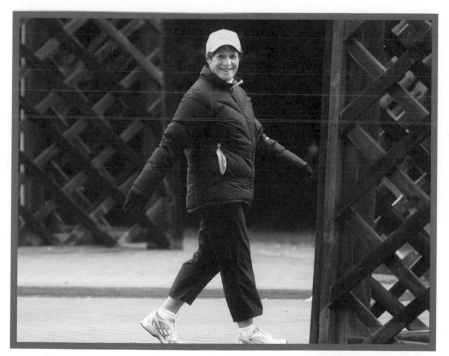

Kuia, Lady Morrison on her daily walk. *Photo Rotorua Post.*

New York had been a long time in the planning and was to be a real high point for Kuia and friends. Not shy of publicity, she wanted to make sure others heard about it, and particularly wanted their story to inspire others and to be told back home. A television crew followed Team Lady Morrison Marathoners in their spunky hot-pink Ts, tracking them through the build-up and capturing those moments of elation when they made it to the finish line. The folks back home heard about these women all right.

Kuia may have been the oldest, but there was no mistaking who was leading this team as they prepared for the big day, very, very early and well before daybreak on a freezing winter morning. An experienced hand, she was well planned and equipped, because she knew all about the cold and taxing discomfort of the pre-race routine and build-up to start time. The girls would be thanking her later that day for all the gear they had to keep warm — sleeping bags, blankets and a blow-up mattress should any of the team need to crash on something soft! Or just sit down at some point on a very big day out.

The marathons have been a highlight for her, and she says she has loved the social contact and the camaraderie that come with getting a team to marathons — and home again to tell a happy tale.

But her more modest walks and her encouragement of local women around Rotorua are an everyday part of her life, which she says keep her motivated and bring her satisfaction.

'Doesn't matter whether it's a walk in the park or in Paris. I know most women want to do something that is for themselves. I love helping our Maori women do that. I have the time and the experience to help these young woman just get going and get onto a better path for their health.'

'I'm well known for collecting up women and girls to come and walk with me. I'm not beyond telling them they look like they could do with a really good walk. And I know they see me coming and I know what they think. But that's me. And if I can help teach any woman to look after her body, I'm happy with that.'

She may have slowed down a little, but weekends still call for a very respectable walking effort. Often with a fellow walker, but sometimes alone, she regularly does a three-hour round trip out to Rotorua airport and back. And she always sets a cracking pace, according to the many who have walked with her.

'I like to walk every day. I need to. I get stroppy if I stay in the house. It's just the way I am, but walking really does it for me.'

PROFILE

Woman on a mission for walking

Steffi Mueller is no stranger to finding motivation and holding onto it in the face of extraordinary odds. The German immigrant has turned her own life experience — and education — to motivating women to get up and get going as though their lives depended on it. In her patch, she has become something of a walking legend over the past decade.

In the 1980s, before the Berlin wall came down, Steffi, with her husband and then tiny daughter, took the brave decision to get out of East Germany and move to West Germany. It took years of struggle and stress for the family to finally get permission to go, and when the word came in November 1988, they had just 24 hours to farewell family and friends and board the train to a new life.

A stint in an immigrant camp followed, then a succession of jobs in West Germany, where they slowly improved their skills and their lot over the next 10 years. For the Muellers, though, New Zealand, with the attractive lifestyle they believed it offered, looked like the place they wanted to make their home.

They set off with two children, no jobs, a modest container of possessions, visitors' visas only, and very little knowledge of the language. Steffi remembers having language books in every room, attending night classes and devouring children's books from the library, to cram her head with the English language. Nevertheless, determination was not enough at first, and she flunked her initial English test. She passed on the second attempt, just a week before the family's visitors' visa was due to expire.

'We faced one problem after the other, but we never gave up.'

Steffi had trained as a chef and today lists university studies in nutrition and weight management plus massage therapy in her resumé. She's also a Nordic walking instructor. From this basket of skills, she has built a career in wellbeing, exercise and motivating others since coming to Mt Maunganui in 1997.

All year round, she's a familiar figure, out walking with her 'charges', encouraging them around the popular Mount walks, up hills and down dales. She's taken her passion public with her own website on motivation, produced a cookbook full of ideas for healthy eating, and mounted a couple of colourful events to promote walking. On New Year's Day, 2008, a good crowd turned out for her first Family Pyjama Beach Walk and she has taken run/walk events as far afield as the challenging Tongariro Crossing. To keep the walking momentum up in her town, she tirelessly distributes leaflets to promote events, secures sponsorship and the support of local media for publicity.

While she wants to get every woman out there walking, she has a focus on helping overweight women with a mixed approach of nutrition, exercise, motivation and support programmes. And she has them on the massage table, too, when a little more nurturing of protesting bodies is in order.

'My passion is to help motivate people and give them their confidence back. To be ready for a healthy lifestyle change, women need to organise their lives to include an exercise programme they will love doing.'

'I help them to set goals for themselves, and I kick butt if they fail to reach them. It is most rewarding to see people whose motto was "I can't", completing triathlons of 5, 10 or 21 kilometres and losing large amounts of weight in the process. I train alongside each one. I want to get them hooked on the benefits. It is important for women to learn to say "no" to some of the demands placed on them and become a little selfish. I like to make them feel special — because they are special — and the change in them after just a few weeks is great to see. Of course it's not just me who notices the big improvements! To make it happen with regular exercise, women need to create their own timetable and book in their own appointment with healthy living.'

On her cheery posts on the Wonder Walkers website, Steffi says to the membership: 'If you need a butt-kicker, just email me and I will take you under my wings.'

Many a local woman may be slimmer, fitter and better off all-round for encountering Steffi, but there have been plenty of benefits for her too as the self-styled mother of local walking women: 'Exercise is a major part of my life every day. It's an essential part of being happy and healthy and it has brought me many treasured friends in this country. And all the positive feedback I get from women makes me happy and keeps me motivated to keep them motivated.'

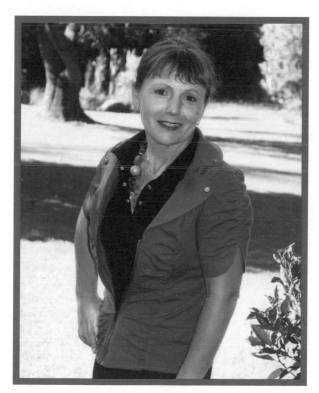

Steffi Mueller.

Chapter 4

GET GOING WITH A WALKING PLAN

To make getting started — and continuing — easier, following a walking plan is a big boost.

Below is a walking plan designed by Wonder Walker's health and fitness expert. It is an introductory walking programme to improve fitness, weight management and health.

The 10k in 10 Weeks Challenge

This is a plan designed to enable beginners and those with a bit more fitness to make a 10-kilometre walk after 10 weeks' training. Follow it, just to get walking and reap the benefits or use this plan to train for your first walking event.

It's a programme with enough variety and intensity to help you stay focused as you feel your fitness improve every week. As you follow this training programme you will be gradually over-loading your heart, lungs and legs over a set period of time in order to improve your fitness. Each week you will be adding extra distance to your longer walk. An increase of around 10 per cent can be tolerated by most beginner walkers each week. Days of training are also matched by some rest days to allow recovery time and physical adaptation.

The programme has two paces: Easy (E) and moderate (M). Those who are a little unfit will want to start on fairly flat terrain. We add in more undulating routes and hill work three weeks into the programme.

Wonder walking week by week

(**M**) — Moderate pace. You should be breathing heavier than normal but able to hold a conversation.

(**E**) — Easy pace. No stopping but walking at a comfortable pace. Go at this pace to recover from a harder session the day before.

A few minutes spent stretching after your training as well as on your 'rest' days will assist your muscle recovery. Include the following muscle groups: hamstrings, quadriceps, calves and upper back/shoulders.

Week 1

Goal: Getting started

Introducing you to three or four walks over your first week.

Day 1: Walk 2 km (E)

Day 2: Walk 2.5 km (M)

Day 3: Rest/stretch

Day 4: Walk day

Day 5: Rest/stretch

Day 6: Walk 5 km (E)

Day 7: Rest/stretch

Week 2

Goal: Staying committed

You may be more tired this week, so the goal is for you to do exactly the same as you did last week but if you only managed three walks last week, try to make it four this week. Any change to daily habits requires a bit of old-fashioned discipline.

Focus on your walking technique. Stay tall. Swing your arms rhythmically and roll your foot through from heel to toe. Tighten your abdominals and your butt muscles as well. Breathe deeply. If you were very low in fitness when you started last week, take an extra rest day if you need to this week.

Week 3

Goal: To keep building your stamina

Adding in some small hills to your terrain this week increases strength in your legs and arms. The extra effort the hills require will also boost your cardiovascular fitness. If you feel in need of extra recovery this week, substitute one walk with a swim.

Day 1: Walk 4 km (M)

Day 2: Walk 3 km (M)

Day 3: Rest/stretch

Day 4: Walk 3 km (E **)

Day 5: Walk 2 km (M)

Day 6: Walk 6 km (E, hilly)

Day 7: Rest/stretch

** Add mixed terrain here — flat to start with, then add some gentle hills.

Week 4

Goal: To add in one longer walk to 'over-load' your body even more

This week is a tough one but your efforts will force your cardiovascular system to work even harder. This is the way to improved fitness.

Day 1: Walk 4 km (M)

Day 2: Walk 5 km (M)

Day 3: Rest/stretch

Day 4: Walk 6 km (E)

Day 5: Walk 4 km (M)

Day 6: Rest /stretch

Day 7: Walk 8 km (E)

Week 5

Goal: Have a recovery week — you've reached the halfway mark

This week we have extra rest days and/or cross training such as swimming or cycling. The focus is to allow your body to adjust and recover from the extra demands being placed on it. It's now time to review progress and your nutrition. In the next training weeks you will need to increase your fluid intake and make sure you have good quality food 1–2 hours before your longer walks.

Day 1: Rest (or easy swim)

Day 2: Walk 5 km (M)

Day 3: Rest/stretch

Day 4: Walk 4 km (E)

Day 5: Walk 5 km (M)

Day 6: Rest/stretch

Day 7: Swim or cycle, 20–30 mins (E)

Week 6

Goal: Start adding in some extra distance

Day 1: Walk 5 km (M)

Day 2: Rest/stretch

Day 3: Walk 4 km (M)

Day 4: Walk 5 km (E)*

Day 5: Rest/stretch

Day 6: Walk 8 km (E-M)

Day 7: Rest/stretch

*If you are entering an event, try to complete this session over the course if you can.

Week 7

Goal: Keep building speed and stamina by covering longer distances in a shorter time

Day 1: Walk 5 km (E)

Day 2: Walk 3 km (M)

Day 3: Rest/stretch

Day 4: Walk 8 km (M)*

Day 5: Walk 2 km (E)

Day 6: Walk 5 km (M)

Day 7: Rest/stretch

*If you are training for an event, complete this session at the pace you want to do on the actual day of the event. If possible, walk today on the event course.

Week 8

Goal: Keep building your distance

If you are training for an event, try to focus on going faster. The longer walks this week are designed to be a psychological boost so you know that you can do it on event day. This week, we include some hill walking to consolidate the strength you have been gaining.

Day 1: Walk 8 km (E/M)

Day 2: Walk 3 km (M)

Day 3: Rest/swim/stretch

Day 4: Walk 10 km (E)

Day 5: Rest/stretch

Day 6: Walk 6 km (E/M)

Day 7: Rest/stretch

The last two weeks have seen a big increase in the total distance walked. Make sure you have the time to do the longer distances at your own pace. Slow walkers should carry extra water/glucose drink or fruit for added energy on day 4, when you do the 10-kilometre distance.

Week 9

Goal: Fine-tuning and consolidating

Same programme as last week but add two more kilometres on to your long walk. This is known as 'over distance' training, ensuring you can go the distance if you have an event coming up. Practise the timing of food and fluid intakes on the long walks.

Day 1: Walk 8 km (E)

Day 2: Walk 3 km (M)

Day 3: Rest/swim/stretch

Day 4: Walk 12 km (E/M)

Day 5: Rest/stretch

Day 6: Walk 5 km (E/M)

Day 7: Rest

Week 10

Goal: Taper off and prepare to feel refreshed if you are competing in an event.

Day 1: Walk 8 km (E)

Day 2: Walk 5 km (E)

Day 3: Rest/stretch

Day 4: Walk 5 km (E)

Day 5: Rest/stretch

Day 6: Walk 4 km (E)

Day 7: 10 km Event

By now you should be a new woman. Feeling fit, fabulous and well convinced of the benefits of regular walking.

PROFILE

Three sisters find strength in numbers and in having a plan to follow

A decade ago 54-year-old Sandie decided to take another tack on her battle with weight loss and depression. With around 20 kilograms to lose, she pulled on her shoes and took the first steps towards making walking part of her personal formula for all-round wellbeing. For her, like many other women, getting out the door and talking those first steps was a big challenge.

It has been quite a journey, and she has gathered up other women along the way — including her two older sisters, Lil (57) and Jeannie (59). She was briefly stopped in her tracks by breast cancer and watched the weight piling on again. Today she has refined her own personal walking plan to make sure she has a strategy to keep up the exercise which helps her maintain her health and happiness.

Sandie recognised the barriers to fitting in her daily fix of walking, whether bad weather or personal demands on her time. So she installed a treadmill at home, and every day she is up and walking on it, clocking up a respectable distance before setting off to work and home again — on foot. It takes 30 minutes to walk to work, and she covers 6 kilometres on the round trip. Luckily, her workplace has showers.

She chats, too, to online walking groups of people who are battling weight issues, spurring them on to get active.

Although she changes out of walking gear every day to slip into her role as a call-centre team manager, Sandie has carried her enthusiasm for walking, and its benefits, into the office. She was quick to pull together a team of walkers and inspire them to get out there on a regular schedule, counting steps together.

She says walking with other women has been one of the benefits of her lifestyle. With her two sisters, it is a shared experience that has made a closer bond between the three women in midlife and seen them planning for major walking events together.

'Walking has made such a difference to my life that I tell everyone everywhere. If I inspire one other woman to get walking, it has to be a good thing.'

Chapter 5

WALKING WELL AND PREVENTING INJURIES

If you are serious about getting into walking, it is important to pay attention from the start to how you are walking, the surface you are on, and what you are wearing for the job. Do not forget about hydration or fuel either. While aches and pains could show up, particularly if you are quite unfit, some will be avoided with a bit of correction to your natural technique. While we all have our own distinctive walk, there is more to walking well than just putting one foot in front of the other

Getting your posture right will make a big difference to getting the technique right. You should be standing up tall and straight, keeping your belly button pulled in and your bottom tucked in — as best you can. It may feel strange at first, if you have never paid attention to what is happening around your middle as you walk, but it makes a real difference to getting your core muscles working. And besides, good posture makes you look good.

Then there is the matter of how you propel yourself along with each step. You will get more power if you pay attention to rolling through your step from heel to toe and pushing off from the toes of your back foot. To achieve more power and speed, increase the speed of your steps — not the length of your stride. You'll be slightly rotating your torso as you go, too, which helps to move your arms in time.

Tune up your walking technique

Starting at the top — your head — and working down, following these tips will help you achieve a good walking technique:

head — look ahead, not down, and make sure not to push your neck forward
shoulders — keep them relaxed and not hunched up around your ears
arms — keep them relaxed and close to your body with a bend at the elbow, to help propel you along
back — keep it straight, although you are likely to lean forward a bit on hills
legs — step out and extend them as you walk, but don't take an exaggerated stride.

Thinking about your posture as you set off will remind you to build your technique. It may feel a bit strange at first, but try to keep the key points in mind as you go, noticing the difference it makes to how you are walking.

Getting ready to go — warm up and stretch

Warm up

It is important to warm up before you start exercising — and before you start your stretch routine. Warming up your muscles, and then stretching them, helps make them more flexible and ready for action. This preparation will make walking more comfortable, enhance your range of movement and reduce your chances of injury.

Begin by walking slowly for about five minutes to warm up your body and reduce the risk of straining your muscles or tendons.

In your warm-up routine, you:
• increase your breathing rate
• increase you heart rate
• allow muscles and tendons to stretch
• boost your blood circulation.

Warming down and stretching after your walk helps restore your body to regular activity levels. Giving the muscles a stretch at this point helps release toxins and lactic acid. The general consensus is that it also helps to minimise post walking soreness.

Stretch routine

In a stretch routine, you:
• stretch all your major muscle groups
• stretch gently and slowly
• hold each stretch for at least 15 seconds
• stretch only to where you feel the tension, not pain
• breathe slowly.

In a stretch routine, you use different exercises to stretch the different muscles. Use a kitchen chair if you need support to do these exercises. If you are already outside, a tree, a fence or a buddy will do just as well to support you.

Calf muscles

Step one foot forward and bend the knee while keeping the knee of the back leg straight. Press your back heel down until you can feel a gentle stretch in the calf muscle. Hold this for 20 seconds, and change legs to work the other calf muscle.

Lower calf

Feet on the ground, one leg in front of the other. Bend both knees a little and lean forward. Hold for 20 seconds, then change sides.

Quadriceps

Starting with your feet together. Bend your knee and lift one leg back behind you and grasp it in your hand. Then try drawing your knee and hip back as far as you can. Hold for 20 seconds, then change sides.

Shins

Both feet facing ahead, hands on the back of a chair. Bend both knees a little. Keep front foot on the ground and reach one foot back to rest on your toe as you lean gently forward a little. Hold for 20 seconds, then change sides.

Hips

Feet facing forward with back straight. Gently lower one knee to the ground then lean gently forward. Hold, then change sides.

Hamstrings

Sitting or standing. Extend one leg out with heel to ground. Straighten your knee and bend toes back toward you. Hold, then gently repeat on the other leg.

Warm down

On the homeward stretch, relax and slow your pace in the last five or so minutes of your walk. It is a good idea, too, to repeat some of the stretching you did before you set off.

Aches and pains and injuries

Walking may be easier on the body than running and other high-impact activity, but it can still bring pain and injury, particularly when you step up your activity. Bad posture and inadequate shoes could soon result in problems with knees, feet, hips or your back that could quickly dampen your enthusiasm. Walking is a repetitive exercise, and it will be working certain muscles more than others.

Of course everybody is individual and exercise will have its own sort of impact on each of us. So it is entirely possible that sore knees could become your issue while your buddy is bothered with blisters. Either way, you will both be limping home in pain!

A sudden increase in how far and how fast you walk (tempting if you are the impatient sort who wants results fast) can also cause pain and injury. This is why the experts design walking plans which build distance and speed slowly. An increase of about 10 per cent a week works for most people.

A sensible approach and listening to our bodies suits most people wanting to keep up a regular walking programme. Injury prevention is important and is closely related to how much thought you want to put into protecting yourself and equipping yourself properly. If you are young and fit the prospect of injury may not be top of mind, but the older your body is, the more likely it is that bits of you will be more worn than others. Sometimes the pain hits before you see it coming when you start to do something different, putting new demands on your body.

What to do when things start to hurt

When things start to hurt it is unwise to ignore it. The first line of defence is to stop and rest, and apply ice or something cold to the sore spot.

If you are committed to walking, take time to check out what is causing the pain and what your options are other than giving up. You may go straight to your doctor, a physiotherapist or your massage therapist, but you can also check out the range of self-help products now available over-the-counter to sportspeople, from special support gear and orthotics for your shoes, to balms and rubs, and of course anti-inflammatory medications. Any one of these or a combination may well take care of your problems. Of course you may be opposed to taking medications in any circumstances, but if you do want to try them you will need to note the cautions on the anti-inflammatory packet, or talk to an expert first.

There is a huge range of products out there to target and prevent injury, so it is well worth knowing if any would be effective in making walking easier for you. One small thing can make a big difference — from socks to salves!

For distance walker Tanja, the discovery of a technically advanced skin lubricant made a huge difference to her comfort and post walk condition: 'I used to be chafed raw in many spots until I found this stuff. I don't know why I had never heard of it — I guess I never went looking for something to prevent chafing. Chafing is a real problem if you are a bigger woman.

Using this lubricant has made a huge difference. So have my sports bra and my technical walking socks with the separate toe partitions. They stop my toes rubbing together.'

Walking surfaces can contribute to injury, too. Walking on concrete is particularly hard on the body, and the angles of hills and beaches bring their own pressures.

Happy feet

Having shoes that are right for the shape of your feet and good socks are a good start in keeping your feet in shape for walking (see the section on choosing footwear). For extra support, though, you may want to insert an orthotic into your shoes. You can buy orthotics over-the-counter, but getting them customised to your feet may give the best results. They will make a real difference if your feet roll in (which is known as 'over-pronation') or you need extra arch support. Over-pronation is common enough, but the impact of the foot roll not only twists the foot, it also pulls on the knee and shin, potentially causing pain up through those areas. Pretty soon this common scenario could slow you down unless countered with effective support.

Common complaints

The following are common complaints among walkers.

Blisters: Even with the best gear, sore feet are the things that bring many a walker to a halt, particularly over longer distances. The inevitable rubbing of your feet by both socks and shoes builds up heat and makes your feet more blister-prone. Wearing in new shoes gradually is one line of defence, but there are other lines of attack. You need to keep your feet dry, so experiment with talcum powder or even cornflour. Others favour using a petroleum jelly, such as Vaseline, to prevent friction.

Athlete's foot: It can strike at any time when feet spend long and frequent spells in walking shoes and socks. You will need to get rid of it, so tackle it with persistence according to the instructions given with whatever product you use.

Cracked heels: Painful but they respond well to the application of the specific remedies available over-the-counter to repair them.

Toe nails: They can cause trouble if there is prolonged pressure on them from poorly fitting shoes or when the feet are forced forward in long stretches of downhill walking.

Aching shins: A common bugbear for new walkers putting too much stress on weak shin muscles. A good warm-up helps, but so too does taking a more gradual approach to building up distance. To settle this pain you might need to take a day or two's break from walking and give those legs the RICE treatment: rest, ice, compression, and elevation. Shin pain could also be an issue where a girl's most regular choice of footwear is a pair of high heels!

Knees: Our knees are a hard-working complex of muscles, tendons, and bits and pieces that can get very sore indeed for a host of reasons, including trying to carry too much weight. The good news is that much knee pain and inflammation can be treated at home, without professional intervention. Once again, rest, ice, compression and elevation will help. Pain and anti-inflammatory medication will also help bring things back under control. Massage will also bring relief. Addressing the cause might include a temporary halt in the walking programme while you focus on exercises to build up strength in the sore and troublesome bits.

Chafing: Wherever it occurs it gets worse and worse with a mix of sweat and friction. You can really only deal to it by preventing it from happening in the first place. The problem could be with your choice of walking clothes (see the section on walking gear). Talcum powder or skin gels could also be a wise choice for your anti-chafing weaponry.

Skin trouble: Getting out there presents a big challenge to every woman's complexion. Always protect your skin from sun and weather conditions with good burn protection and moisturising products.

Seeking professional help

Still hurting? Don't give up just because your body is protesting a little or a lot. Call in the experts. Doctors, physiotherapists, massage therapists, podiatrists and personal trainers are only a telephone call away, and have the expertise to get you back in working order. Professional advice can be invaluable when the obstacles seem too big.

Distance-walking newbie Jo Jukes learned the hard way about dealing with pain and getting professional help in the build-up to her 100-kilometre Oxfam Trailwalker challenge: 'I had to work out my approach as I went, making changes and fine-tuning right through my training. I knew I would need good shoes and socks. But I learned the hard way that I needed to get to the physio as soon as anything started to hurt. For me that was always knees and hips, because I had started such a tough schedule without building up enough strength in my legs. I learned the hard way about warming up, stretching and warming down, too! Boy, what a difference doing that made to me the next day. Things didn't hurt half as much.'

Is it time to replace those walking shoes?

Just when you think you have got it all worked out and your body is humming along in great shape, make sure those shoes are keeping up. Once they are starting to wear, toss them out. If they are looking really worn-out, they could already by doing you more harm than good or are likely to start causing trouble soon.

Walking after injury, accident or sickness

Getting successfully back on your feet after injury, surgery, sickness or whatever else has temporarily put you out of action will doubtless be tricky and frustrating. The approach will vary, depending on how major or minor the setback and how long the path to rehabilitation needs to be. Whatever the issues, it is wise to get approval and guidelines from a health and fitness professional before working out a personal plan and programme. Being unrealistic about how long it takes your body to heal, or being too impatient to get right back out there and on track before your body is up to it, could well put you right back on the living-room sofa — tired, sore and disheartened. Or worse, pushing yourself too hard, too soon, could set you further back.

Obviously recovery times and the rebuilding of strength and fitness will vary from one person to another, but having a realistic recovery plan and monitoring your progress will be vital for getting you back on track.

If the injury has been caused by walking, it is essential to know what caused it and to address the underlying problem before trying to crack off at the same pace again. If the problem can be easily put down to tight muscles, lack of stretching, overuse, an old injury, a wonky knee, feet that roll in or out, or shoes that were not up to the task, this is a chance to review your strengths and weaknesses and take stock. A little cross-training (a mix of exercises like cycling, gym work and swimming) that keeps you off your feet, but helps rebuild fitness, could be worth considering in a determined approach to preparing to return to serious walking.

Getting back into your stride could take time, but working out a well-advised plan (rather than relying on optimism and sheer grit) will be essential for a return to happy and beneficial walking.

PROFILE

Struggling into shape for the 100-kilometre Oxfam Trailwalker

She was a bit of a young couch potato, with a few bad habits and no intention of turning into a serious walker, until a bunch of very serious, long-long-distance walkers got her under their spell, nabbing her for one of their very own. Jo Jukes reckons it could have happened to anyone …

Thirty-year-old Jo found herself drawn into serious long-distance walking almost by accident when she took a job as an events team manager with Oxfam, the international agency dedicated to fighting global poverty and injustice.

While the organisation does many things for its cause, Oxfam's annual Trailwalker has become something of a global phenomenon in long-distance walking and running events. It is one of the world's toughest team challenges: every participant must walk a distance of 100 kilometres in 36 hours. The events run in 12 countries and have attracted over 30,000 teams, who between them have walked more than 11 million kilometres, raising in excess of $50 million.

For walkers all over the world, it is a huge challenge on their annual calendars, some returning with their walking buddies looking to better their times or just to do it again. Not surprisingly it is widely acknowledged — from the fittest participants to the newbies — as a life-changing experience in many, many ways. Some even take it on more than once in a year, travelling to other countries to do so. There is a big team of professionals and volunteers working all year round to make this event the success it has become.

The challenge takes place in New Zealand in April, when the teams gather, along with piles of gear and food, teams of well-wishers and crowds of supporters. Typically they have trained together for many months, forming strong bonds and friendships along the way. Not everyone makes it to the finish of course, but for so many that do, it is the beginning of a whole new chapter in their commitment to and interest in fitness, and embracing the kind of challenge that has taken them way out of their comfort zone.

There are countless inspiring stories from the participants of all ages, shapes and sizes, from all walks of life, about what taking part has meant for them and what they have learned about themselves — and their bodies. Doing the Oxfam is an achievement of which they can be very proud. The post-event proliferation of tales and photographs says it all, and hooks in many new participants every year.

For the 2011 New Zealand event challenge there were 300 teams, or 1200 people, registered. Among them were plenty others like Jo — somehow they had just found themselves in the company of mad keen Trailwalker veterans and got caught up in the fervour of it all. All through the summer and winter these teams are out nights and weekends, pushing themselves on a training schedule of quite gruelling preparation, building stamina, planning menus, and making sure they have the sponsorship in place that will be their contribution to the fund-raising side of things.

As the manager of marketing events for Oxfam in New Zealand, Jo thought she would have to literally 'walk the talk' and join staff when they first floated the idea of entering the challenge themselves. At that stage they were only months out from the next event. Unlike the fit, competitive distance walkers who are well practised in preparing for such daunting challenges, Jo was many, many steps away from being a serious walker. In May 2010, Jo's team made the decision to enter the Sydney race in the last weekend of August and immediately started on the tough training schedule that would see them all finish together just a few months later in Australia.

And while Jo says she won't be taking on such a huge challenge again in a hurry, doing the Oxfam was certainly a huge satisfaction and a saga she will never forget. These days, she has always got another event coming up on her calendar: 'It gives me something to aim for. It keeps me going.'

Before the challenge, walking had mostly consisted of exercising the short legs of her two dogs Euan (a West Highland terrier) and Phoebe (a little Maltese/Shih Tzu-cross) who went with her on regular ambles in a local park. Life even changed for the pets during the rigorous training regime, when the two small dogs sometimes found themselves caught up in the dramatically stepped-up exercise routine. Euan, never a big walker, got up to around seven kilometres, and Phoebe was running 20 kilometres on training days.

With not many months to prepare for the challenge, Jo's team figured out some clever strategies to get them going and keep them going, actively seeking opportunities to propel themselves into a daunting training regime without having to work out all of their own schedules and routes from scratch. Often they went where others were going or had gone before them.

First off, they committed themselves to being the 'tail-end Charlies' in scheduled winter weekend off-road races, and were therefore pledged to following the stragglers home over the course. Attaching themselves to existing events to put them in the company of others with big walking goals helped keep motivation up. All this had to be built in and coped with around a busy working week, other life commitments, and things like running a home. Having supportive partners and friends was critical in both a psychological and a practical sense.

They walked by day and night over marked bush trails and through forests, Jo tripping frequently in the dark (and sometimes spooky) bush when fatigue or hunger saw her forgetting to lift her feet: 'I was the weakest link. If I got too tired or hungry and started tripping over, the others would tell me to have something to eat and lift my feet! If I didn't lift my feet, I fell over.'

On many Friday nights they set out on a 15-kilometre walk, returned to base to eat, then headed back out to keep walking, building fitness and distance and the all-important resolve that could be more fragile on some days than others, particularly if you were new to it. Jo's teammates knew what they were in for and knew how to pace themselves, but time was short and Jo had to learn — and suffer — as she trained. Strain, pain and learning how to deal with it were part of the price as she figured out what would over-tax her body, or worse, knock her out of the team altogether.

On many winter nights, while their friends were holed up in cosy houses, Jo and her teammates were out in all weathers building up the kilometres. In addition to hooking up with group events, they had their own routes for team trainings. Their weekend walks took them all over the region and further afield, over mixed and tricky terrain. One weekend in late May they did a 16-kilometre cross-country walk. In June they undertook a coastal walk between two popular, wild beaches. With the race day coming up fast in the last weekend of July, they did a big circuit of 63.2 kilometres on an island, keeping up an average pace of 5 kilometres an hour. They were on the move for 12 hours 40 minutes and stopped for just 1 hour 30 minutes. The log for the Friday night first segment of the walk went like this:

Friday night:
Distance: 26.4 km
Time: 5 hrs 40 min moving, 40 min stopped
Moving average: 4.7 km per hour
Vertical climb: 1010 metres
Terrain: trails and roads
Weather: Clear

By this stage, Jo was well into the training for a huge walk, but she was feeling it and was by no means confident. A knee injury from childhood added to her difficulties.

Jo recalls being very excited but more than a bit anxious as her team took off for Sydney, and the going was every bit as tough as she knew it was going to be, although she says pulling out was just not an option.

'At first I was very chipper. It sure was a huge struggle in the end. It seemed to go on and on. There were good patches, tough patches, and some very tough patches. I was in pain, I cried, and at one point, around the 70-kilometre mark, I really started to fall apart. It just took everything I had, but it was more than that. It was a real team effort and I could never have done it without them, and all the other people who were willing me on with them. Text messages too, from outside the course, were such a fantastic support to me.'

'I am glad I had the experience and I learned a lot about myself that, without doubt, will stick with me. I also learned a lot about my body and exercise. To do something like this you absolutely have to take it seriously. You have to be in very good shape but you also have to look after your body — willpower and bravado just won't cut it. You need to have good gear and you need to be very well nourished. Hydration is something you can easily forget about, but such a simple thing as having enough to drink is just one of the many things on the list of lessons for newcomers to long-distance walking.'

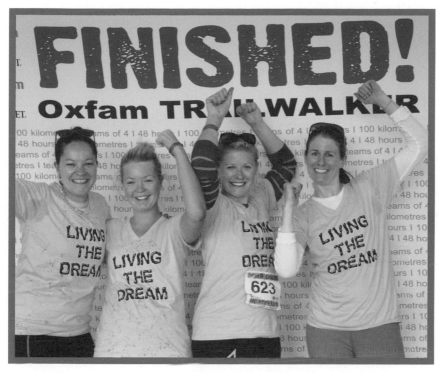

They made it! Oxfam Trailwalker Melbourne, 2011. *Photo Oxfam Australia.*

Chapter 6

GET SMART WITH WALKING TECHNOLOGY: PEDOMETERS AND MOBILE PHONES

Depending on your budget and your comfort level with technology, you can make great use of the simple functions of a pedometer or the new and exciting mobile phone applications for intelligent walking support. Whether it is counting steps or recording a great range of data and sharing it across social networks, there is a tool that will enhance walking for you. Technology could be a girl's best friend when it comes to getting serious about just how much walking you are really doing and if it is enough to be doing good things for your health.

Using a pedometer

The pedometer is a great motivational tool, and investing in one of these clever little things can cost as little as lunch out with a friend. It is a small gadget you wear as you walk that counts your steps.

Sounds so easy, and it is if you are ready to get real about your walking programme and invest in a simple system for keeping track. The tally of your personal efforts will be there for you to count at the end of the day, and record for weeks, months or however long you like. If you take the time to do this, you'll soon have a useful personal log to refer back to whether for motivation or information. The idea of course is that you'll soon be setting goals, reaching them and challenging yourself to increase the distance.

You can buy a good sturdy basic pedometer at most sports stores, but take a while to read the instructions to make sure you are wearing it correctly and it is functioning well, before you set off. It is no use just popping it in your pocket. Clip it securely onto the side of your waistband above your hip, because this is where it can best record those steps and become your faithful secret weapon.

Before you set yourself a target of daily steps, it is wise to use your pedometer (or mobile phone) for about a week to record how many steps you are doing in the normal course of events. Chances are it might be somewhere between 1000 and 3000 if you have a fairly sedentary life and work at a desk job — not as many steps as you may have thought and nowhere near enough to make a difference. If walking is your main exercise, you will need to nearly triple the number of steps you are taking a day to reach the level of exercise that is recommended for wellness.

The experts say that if you fit over 7000 steps and up to 10,000 steps a day into your life, it should be enough to reduce your risk for disease and keep you on the path to a long and healthy life. If you want to lose a significant amount of weight, it is estimated you will need to get up over 12,000 steps a day to achieve that. While you won't have to take that many steps in one burst, a minimum of 6000 steps per walk is said to be the minimum needed to start shifting those kilos. While these quotas vary a bit in the wealth of sources on health and fitness, the variation is not great and you will soon work out how much is far enough for you.

In anyone's book, 10,000 steps is quite a bit of walking! It is about 8 kilometres every day, and quite a big step-up if you are starting from a very sedentary position. It won't happen overnight, but with a plan, and a pedometer, you will be surprised how quickly you can start to increase your number of daily steps.

Keeping an accurate record will take the guesswork out of how well you are doing. Before choosing a pedometer, do a bit of homework and ask for advice. The cheapest will just count your steps, but many now have other features that could make your walking programme more fun, more of a challenge and more interesting. Some of these features include calculating:

• how far you have walked
• how many calories you have burned
• how fast you are walking
• what your pulse rate is.

Different features are important to different people, and if you like a bit of technology you could soon be enjoying learning more about your daily walks. Perhaps you could aim to walk a bit faster for part of your walk or see what hilly stretches do for pulse and calories burned — just some of the options for your to experiment with. Challenge a friend and use your pedometers to work out the rules.

If you are new to walking and not very fit, you might want to start off with modest increases and increase the number of daily steps by around 20 per cent a day for the first week. Aim for the same increase the next week, and again the following week. Remember, you do not have to make it happen all at once, and a couple of weeks into using the pedometer you will find yourself looking for other chances during your day to add to that tally of steps and reach the total you are aiming for.

There are so many ways to build the time you spend moving about every day: Get yourself into the swing of thinking 'more steps' by:

• parking a bit further from your destination
• taking a brief walk at lunchtime
• taking the stairs instead of the lift
• walking to the corner store
• making an extra circuit or two of the shopping mall
• walking the dog a bit more often.

Keeping a record of your steps, and seeing how far you have come, will help keep up the motivation. This could be a simple handwritten record of steps each day, but could also include the route taken, the time, and your speed plus any notes (for example, hill sections added in, variations on the route).

Soon enough you will have committed to memory how many steps these little extra steps you take are adding to your daily total and you won't have to rely on your pedometer to tell you when you are meeting your goals. Within a month, many people find they are doing 10,000 steps.

Thousands of people have made pedometers a great little friend rather than a pocket tyrant once they have become accustomed to using them as a tool to get into walking as a serious form of exercise. And the many organisations that have introduced the eight-week workplace 10,000-step programmes have reported many benefits, with healthier and fitter staff who are happier and more productive at work — and call in sick a lot less often.

Tips for success with a pedometer

- Buy a reputable brand.
- Buy one that is easy to use.
- Consider the features that would be best for you.
- Wear it correctly.
- Keep a log of your progress.
- Set realistic goals and build on them.
- Reward yourself for achieving your goals.

Keeping a walking log

A walking log could be a very simple chart made up for weeks in advance, allowing for more or less emphasis on the things that matter to you, such as performance, weight loss, increasing your hill work, avoiding dodgy terrain, lonely spots, or too many steep steps.

	Distance	Speed	Time	Notes (route, weather, hills, hazards, etc)
Monday				
Tuesday				
Wednesday				
Thursday				
Friday				
Saturday				
Sunday				

Utilising mobile-phone walking applications

For the techno fans and girls who won't go far without their phones, there is another good reason for taking the mobile along, besides staying in touch, listening to stuff, and cruising around the net on a solo coffee stop.

Applications for mobile phones like 'map my walk' are relatively new, but they have been quickly adopted by walkers who are up with technology and like to interface on exercise challenges with like-minded friends on social networks from Facebook to Twitter.

Since mobile-phone walking applications were introduced in very recent years, they have been so regularly updated that their features, benefits and capabilities change all the time. There are walking applications available for all types of mobile phone which can be downloaded free in a heartbeat. And there is no stopping to fumble because you operate the system as you walk by earphone remotes.

In a nutshell, these mobile phone 'apps' enable you to use the GPS function in your phone to track and record your fitness activity. You can record times, distance, speed, pace, calories burned, and the route you have travelled.

You can save all this information and upload it to websites and share it with others. You can map your routes, and create graphs and calendars. If you like, you can add in a sort of virtual walking buddy by configuring regular announcements through your earphones, giving you announcements on things like time, distance and performance. You can communicate progress as you go, and keep track of others.

Using walking 'apps' on a late-model phone may be a much more expensive and time-consuming way to go than using a simple pedometer, but it certainly takes the simple activity of walking to another level. Not only can you collect an overwhelming amount of data, but you can also transport yourself into a sort of mobile walking community, both as you go and after the event. No wonder the new generation of walkers doesn't leave home without their phones!

PROFILE

Louise Shanly:
a pedometer and an office walking programme

In a way, a successful strategy for walking and weight control came to Louise at her office desk when she was coming up to her 50th birthday.

Louise was no stranger to struggling with significant weight problems, which she had battled with formidable stints of running and walking over the years, but the weight always crept up again when her vigilance and discipline waned. She had been diagnosed with Type 1 diabetes in her 20s, and in the following decades she had tried with mixed success to deal with these issues while juggling child-rearing, work and running her home.

In her mid-40s, over a six-month period, she had managing to lose an astonishing 22 kilograms — about a kilogram a week — by stepping up her efforts to run every day and by nearly halving what she ate. The running was doing the trick, but knee problems forced her to quit and soon enough her weight began creeping up again.

Fortunately, the opportunity to make a fresh start came in the form of the work-based 10,000 steps a day programme. She seized the chance to sign up, and strapped on the pedometer, thereby locking her into doing her daily quota of steps. She has taken part in the annual exercise challenges ever since she joined the business, where she is a facilitator and trainer. But more importantly, the first challenge brought back the awareness of all the benefits of exercise and gave her the motivation to get back into a walking regime all year round.

'It got me going again. I feel pretty good and I can't believe how much more energy the exercise gives me, and I always get a real boost from the endorphin rush at the end of every good walk. It has also been very good for controlling my diabetes.

'I know it's the maintenance programme that is the answer for keeping me well, happy, and keeping my weight and my diabetes under control. I had to learn to take a long-term view of the role exercise would need to play in my life, and learn how to build it into my day in a way that would work for me. There are no excuses anymore — I am now totally committed to taking responsibility for that.'

'It hasn't always been easy, and there have been times when it would have been so tempting to give in and give up. To come home after a day at work and do something else. Ghastly weather or many other things could easily distract me, but it's much easier now that I have made walking part of every day and been able to stick with it. I accept that it is just what I do. It is what I have to do. If I don't do it, I feel out of sorts. It doesn't matter whether I am home or away, or what the weather is doing. My friends and family know that every evening, wherever I am, I come in, I get changed, and I go straight out again for my walk of about 40 minutes. Of course, having a very supportive husband makes it easier to take that time out for myself. I am highly motivated and I know that I won't break my commitment to my routine.'

As well as taking her daily evening walk around the waterfront (wet, dry, windy or dark), Louise also makes sure she takes many extra steps during the day by stepping out from her desk at lunchtimes and by always taking the stairs. 'Those things are just a habit now. And you know that once it all becomes a habit rather than a chore, you are on your way.'

Over the years Louise has learned a few of the tricks she needed to get out walking and to ensure she keeps it up. She realised the pedometer challenge could be her kick-start, providing the ready-made programme and group support that have helped many others to get going. Enlisting social and family support to back her and to give her space enabled her to keep up her walking. She also invested in relatively expensive walking gear that is comfortable, functional and makes her feel good. Making that outlay, she says, is part of making a serious commitment to walking. She also worked out the time of day in a busy schedule that she could realistically put a ring around as 'my time' and be sure she could routinely head out the door without any pressure from other demands.

These are her tips for a successful walking programme:

- Take a long-term view and aim to make it a habit.
- Invest in good shoes, socks and walking clothes that you enjoy changing into.
- Get family support.
- Choose a time of day to walk that suits your lifestyle and do not waiver from it.
- Take responsibility for your routine and make no excuses.

Chapter 7

ABOUT NUTRITION, WALKING AND WEIGHT LOSS

Exercise and diet are inextricably linked in the management of our weight and overall health. We need to work on both things together, because the sad reality is that a girl would have to walk an awfully long way indeed to keep the kilos off if she's regularly overeating and downing several glasses of wine every night.

Most of us, say the experts, fall into the trap of underestimating how much we are eating, and overestimating how much we are exercising. And it is that little fib to ourselves that makes it hard to lose weight and to keep it off!

It is a well-known fact, too, that although many people take up walking to control their weight, many of them are hoping for a miracle without facing up to what they are scoffing down on a regular basis. If that is the case, the result of all their activity is invariably disappointing.

Wendy Sweet and Christel Dunshea-Mooij are two fit and healthy experts in the science of eating and exercise. Both are advisors to women at www.wonderwalkers.com, where they share their well-founded, sound advice.

Christel Dunshea-Mooij (MSc Nutrition, Hons) is a performance nutrition expert who has heard every story in the book about battling the bulge and the barriers people put up to sensible eating, but she says it is never too late to start turning things around: 'A few little changes begin to make a bit of difference. And that's okay to start with.' Nevertheless, it is a change of approach to the way we eat that will make for weight loss and control, rather than an obsession with numbers and measurements.

'It's no use kidding yourself,' says Christel. 'After a big meal of fish and chips you'd have to walk 33 kilometres to work it off!' Oh dear. But she says it is also the same daunting picture for trying to walk off the smaller transgressions.

Burning off calories

What it really takes to burn off those 'treats'

1 x croissant	23g fat — 11km
50g bag of chips	18g fat — 7000 steps
1 x meat pie	24g fat — 11km
1 x sausage roll	23g fat — 11 km
1 small hamburger + reg fries	28g fat — 11km
1 x battered fish + chips	63g fat — 33km

And there's more. Christel says it takes 82 minutes to walk off your average muesli bar, and about an hour and a half of walking to use up the unwanted calories from a can of coke. But as she says, there is no need to get bogged down by numbers. Everyone wants a treat; they just need to remember that it comes with a price. 'Occasional' is the operative word.

Making small, gradual changes is the easiest way to change your diet, as you give yourself time to get used to a change before introducing another one. You also need to allow yourself a treat now and then, and not feel bad when life gets in the way. But, if weight control is your goal, then you need to get back to making healthy eating choices the next day or you are not going to make much progress.

The best approach to maintaining a healthy weight is to adopt a healthy lifestyle. Limit alcohol intake, and give your body all that it needs from each of the four food groups daily. Cut back on fatty, salty and sugary foods, and drink plenty of liquids, especially water, every day.

Food groups and recommended intakes

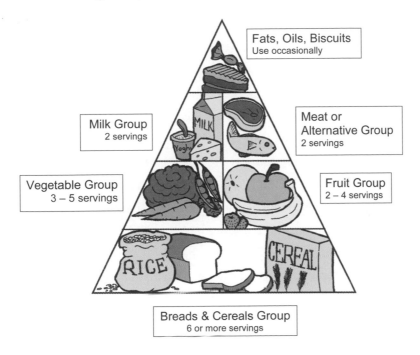

These are the food groups and the recommended daily intakes:
• fruit and vegetables: 5 + servings
• bread and cereals: 6 servings
• meat, fish and alternatives:1 to 2 servings
• milk and diary: 3 servings

Where calories lurk

Until quite recently some people thought that it was carbohydrate intake that was making us fat. In fact, it is the amount of calories (from fat, carbohydrate and protein) that have a direct bearing on the weight we carry. So keeping our weight under control means trying to avoid foods with a higher energy density and higher calorie count.

Energy density of foods

Energy density is the ratio of calories to the actual weight of your food. Therefore, a food that is of high energy density provides a large amount of calories in a small weight, while a food of low energy density has fewer calories for the same weight. In other words, just a few mouthfuls of a favourite food (alas!) can pack a big calorie punch. Foods can vary enormously in energy density. For the same number of calories you can eat just a quarter of a cup of raisins compared with two cups of grapes.

Many studies have shown that people eat the same weight of food daily, no matter what the calorie count. This shows that the energy density of foods affects satiety. You may think you don't have more on your plate than your friend, but the calorie count could be far higher — at every meal.

It is handy to know that water added to food provides a more satisfying portion and lowers the energy density of any food (chocolate vs chocolate milk, for example). You can often lower the energy of favourite recipes by simply adding naturally water-rich vegetables. When you do this, you can eat more for the same number of calories or eat your usual portion and take in fewer calories.

Healthy meals

Aim to fill half of your plate with vegetables, a quarter of your plate with low glyceamic index (GI) carbohydrates, and the other quarter with lean protein, such as fish, lean meat and legumes.

Use water-rich foods to lower the energy density of your meals

- Eat fruit with breakfast — half a grapefruit, an orange, an apple or a small banana.
- Top cereals, pancakes and wholegrain toast with fruits such as peaches, blueberries, strawberries or raspberries.
- For a snack, choose fresh fruit rather than dried fruit or baked or fried food. Add vegetables such as courgettes, peppers, onion, aubergine and

spinach to pasta dishes and pizza. Add extra salad vegetables to sandwiches.
- Increase the proportion of vegetables in stir-fry dishes, soups and stews.
- Include a green salad or a fruit salad with dinner, and choose desserts that include fruit.
- Be aware that it is more satiating when water is incorporated into a food than when the water is consumed separately as a drink. This is why when you drink a glass of low-fat milk or a smoothie, or eat a bowl of soup, you are not hungry for a while. However, this is not the case with cordials, juices and carbonated sodas.

Take a positive approach to weight management and try to lower the overall energy density of your diet. This is a lot more fun than trying to squeeze the fat and sugar out of every morsel you put in your mouth. And it is an easy change to make that can soon become a way of life.

'It is very important not to become obsessed about what you eat, and these days we have moved away from setting specific quantities as guidelines. Nevertheless, we live in an age of super-sized servings and we are piling food onto much bigger plates and bowls than our parents used,' says Christel. 'Just being aware of these things can help us in our mealtime choices without making too much fuss about what we eat.'

Fuelling that morning walk

Whether you should eat breakfast before or after your morning walk depends on your goals. If your goal is to improve your performance, have something to eat before you start out. But if you want to lose weight, and you will do the same amount of exercise on an empty stomach, do not have breakfast until after your walk.

Exercising in a fasted state (eight hours since you had dinner or an evening snack) is said to be more efficient from a fat-burning perspective. It results in a greater proportion of fat being used as the fuel for your walk, compared to doing the same walk after a breakfast containing carbohydrates. However, you will more likely be able to exercise harder and for a longer period if you have had a light breakfast before your morning walk.

Personally, when I try to walk without having breakfast, I feel wobbly, I don't seem to have any stamina and my pace is slow. But 30 minutes to an hour after breakfast I am ready to walk anywhere at a steady pace!

A breakfast for walking

Breakfast eaten before exercise is only useful once it has been digested and absorbed. This means you need to time your food intake so that the fuel becomes available during the exercise period. The time needed for digestion depends on the type and quantity of food consumed. Generally, foods higher in fat, protein and fibre tend to take longer to digest than other foods. Large quantities of foods take longer to digest than smaller quantities. You need to experiment to find the timing that best suits your individual needs.

Breakfast before your morning walk (if you are choosing to fuel for performance) should provide sufficient amounts of carbohydrate, fluid, and a little protein, and should be low in fat. It is useful to consider other nutritional goals, too, and opt for a breakfast that also provides a wide variety of nutrients, including vitamins and minerals, such as fruit and vegetables.

The following are some healthy options for breakfast:
• wholegrain toast plus a poached egg and a grilled tomato
• wholegrain toast spread with 2 tablespoons of avocado, a tomato and a pot of yoghurt
• wholegrain bread roll with low-fat cheese plus fruit
• raisin bread, plus pot of yoghurt
• fruit salad with yoghurt
• fruit smoothie made with a cup of low-fat milk, a cup of fruit and 2 tablespoons yoghurt (optional: add Weet-bix or half a cup of oats)
• allbran with low-fat milk and fruit
• rolled oats with low-fat milk and fruit.

Foods with a low glycaemic index (GI) are better

Foods with carbs have different effects on blood glucose levels. Foods with a low GI cause a slower, sustained release of glucose to the blood, whereas foods with a high GI cause a rapid, short-lived rise in blood glucose. It is therefore suggested that your blood glucose levels will be better sustained during your walk by low glycaemic index carbohydrates.

Don't forget about hydration

We need plenty of fluids, and conventional wisdom tells us that eight glasses a day — most of which should be water — will keep us hydrated. Starting the day by drinking a glassful is a good habit. On this basis, if you're walking for an hour or less you're likely to be well enough hydrated. However, if you are off on a longer walk your water needs will have to be worked on according to your weight, the environment and the walking challenge ahead. Christel suggests using the simple chart below to help you keep an eye on how hydrated you are and to work out what to take into account. Light-coloured urine shows you are well hydrated, but dark urine is a sure sign you need another drink – now! The darker shading in the chart indicates whether you are *likely* or *very likely* to need water. If you are new to walking distances, you'll need to make a hydration plan of your own.

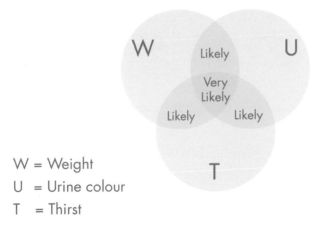

W = Weight
U = Urine colour
T = Thirst

Eating and burning up calories

Wendy Sweet says research shows that when we get the right balance between the calories we eat and how many of them we use up, our weight stays stable. She explains it like this on the Wonder Walkers website:

$$\text{energy balance} = \text{energy intake} + \text{energy output}$$
$$\text{(our weight)} = \text{(what we eat)} + \text{(what we sweat out)}$$

It sounds so simple, so why then do some women seem to lose weight or put it on so much more easily than their friends? Science has given us some of the answers, and it is an issue of great interest to health and weight researchers, so we are not alone in the battle to figure it out.

Energy balance is a basic equation, but it is useful to go into the subject in a bit more depth, in order to really understand the basis of weight loss and — all importantly — how it might, or might not, work out for you. Features which all play a huge part in being able to control your weight include genetics, your resting metabolism, your level of activity, and the quality and quantity of your food intake.

Total daily energy expenditure (TDEE) is the term used to describe how much energy is used by an individual during a 24-hour period. TDEE is made up of three primary components:
• resting metabolic rate (RMR)
• the thermic (heat generating) effects of exercise and physical activity (TEPA)
• the thermic effects of feeding (TEF).

Therefore, the equation underlying the energy balance equation is:

$$\text{TDEE} = \text{RMR} + \text{TEPA} + \text{TEF}$$

It might sound confusing, but understanding this formula will help you lose weight, advises Wendy Sweet. It breaks down as follows.

Resting metabolic rate (RMR)

Your metabolic rate at rest accounts for 60 per cent to 70 per cent of all calories burning in the body. Resting metabolic rate (RMR) refers to the amount of energy required and used by the body to maintain organ systems and body temperature. Because muscle tissue is the largest tissue in the entire body, there is now a lot of interest in how RMR can be manipulated upwards through the development of more muscle. In other words, by building muscle your metabolism increases, which helps burn calories.

If you grow and tone muscles by overloading them, they become more active metabolically. This means that when you are at rest, maybe just sitting on the sofa, you will burn more calories if you have more muscle on your body.

Adding resistance training into your schedule helps prevent the loss of the muscle tissue you already have. This is even more important as we age.

Thermic effects of exercise and physical activity (TEPA)

Structured exercise (such as walking for 60 minutes) and non-structured activity (such as housework) account for more calories burnt. In fact, most research shows that 15 to 30 per cent of total daily energy expenditure is accounted for by the energy required for structured and unstructured daily exercise.

This is another reason why health messages targeting those who do not do any structured activity concentrate on 'snack-tivity' — that is, activity which responds to daily lifestyles, like walking to work, doing housework, washing the car, etc.

This non-structured movement has been given the acronym NEAT. It stands for Non-exercise Activity Thermogenesis and is the increase in temperature we gain from our lifestyle activity, which in turn influences our metabolic rate.

Turning up the intensity of your planned workouts contributes to greater TEPA. You will burn more calories by exercising more vigorously about two days a week. Your internal metabolic rate will remain higher after a more energetic workout because this has elevated your heart rate, blood pressure and temperature.

Even better, if you do your structured exercise (daily walk) first thing in the morning, your metabolism stays elevated for as long as the non-structured effect of activity kicks in. It is all about intensity of effort, and this is what inevitably gets great weight loss results in the longer term.

Thermic effect of feeding (TEF)

The final component in the energy expenditure equation relates to food: what we eat, when we eat and how much we eat.

The thermic effect of feeding (TEF) refers to the energy required for the digestion, absorption, transport, metabolism (energy transfer) and storage of consumed food. In other words, it is the internal energy required to convert the muffin you eat into energy for movement. Or, if you are not moving much, to convert the components of the muffin (fatty acids and glucose) into fat storage areas.

This act of converting the food we eat into either energy or storage accounts for approximately 10 to 15 per cent of daily calories burned. It is also the rationale behind the fact that people who do not eat much (for example, who go on extreme diets or very low-calorie diets) are actively slowing down their metabolism.

To speed up metabolism — eat little and often!

When life just gets in the way

Throughout our life stages, a host of factors influence our metabolism and potential for weight fluctuations. Apart from pregnancy, weight change with aging is perhaps the influence that people see and feel the most. Increasing age equates to decreasing RMR as people generally become less active. Physical inactivity contributes to a loss of muscle over time, and it is to this aspect that researchers attribute an additional drop of RMR of 2 to 3 per cent. This decrease can be minimised as we continue to age, though. Walking and regular resistance training work wonders.

And finally, we cannot discuss metabolic rate and calorie-burning without mentioning some specific hormones. For those people under stress — including those with poor sleep patterns and insomnia — weight loss becomes harder. Adrenaline, the stress hormone, becomes elevated, and over time another hormone, cortisol, kicks in when stress levels go into overdrive for long periods of time. This hormone very simply encourages the body to retain fat stores rather than use fat for energy. It is a complex issue, but getting off the stress wagon, getting good quality sleep as well as eating fruit and veggies to get vital antioxidants are still the best undisputed strategies for building resilience, boosting metabolism and maintaining energy for life.

Walk for weight loss — getting your heart rate up

Intensity is the factor to building fitness and making those kilos start to melt away. You have to walk at a purposeful, brisk pace — breathing moderately hard and still able to talk — but fast enough to get your heart rate up. And you will need to do this regularly and sustain the pace throughout most of your walk. For beginner walkers, the recommended level is at a heart rate of between 50 and 70 per cent. You can calculate this by checking your pulse once you have been walking for a while, or use a pedometer or heart-rate monitor to tell you how hard you are working.

Of course you will need to warm up to avoid making the mistake of many a zealous new walker who tries to go too far too fast. Once you are walking for at least 30 minutes at a good pace without stopping, and doing this at least four to five times a week, you will start to see results.

Take it slowly at first if you have to, but sticking with it will soon bring sufficiently pleasing progress to spur you on into better shape. If it has worked for thousands of other women, it will work for you, too.

PROFILE

A change of tack on weight management

At about 93 kilograms on a 1.52 m (5 feet 3 inches) frame, Tanja took on the 100-kilometre Oxfam Trailwalker challenge in 2009. She gave it her best on the day, but she had to pull out at the 88-kilometre mark. She says that missing by 12 kilometres 'haunted' her for the next two years.

Tanja had been keen on distance walking for a while before she entered the event, but weight loss or weight control at that stage had not been a motivator. Rather, she loved walking and how it made her feel; she loved the challenge of it.

While she may have lost a few kilograms from her first Trailwalker, her long and regular training walks were having little impact on her weight. Tanja says she had been overweight for much of her life, and in her own words 'used to have an unhealthy relationship with dieting and food'.

Training for and participating in that first long-distance walk was a great achievement for the then 36-year-old, but it was being short of the finish line by 12 kilometres that sprang to mind whenever she thought about the event.

After the 2009 Trailwalker she admitted to herself that carrying the extra weight had probably been a significant factor in her failure to finish. 'Despite believing strongly in the concept of health at every size, I had to accept that losing some of that weight might have made the all-important difference between not making it and being able to finish.'

Determination to compete in the Trailwalker again and to finish it became a turning point in her thinking about diet and food. She says the fuel she would require for her training forced her to plan a healthy eating plan rather than an unhealthy diet.

When she took off two years later in April 2011 on her second Trailwalker attempt, she had addressed the demon of eating issues and had lost 18 kilograms over as many months, weighing in at around 75 kilograms.

The weight loss, she says, did make a difference to her performance, and her team finished in 30.5 hours.

Being part of the Wonder Walkers online community of walking women has been part of her successful strategy to keep going and keep challenging herself with major walking events. And to keep up the work with weight control.

'I went looking for an online community of walkers because I guess I wanted to hang around with people who understood why I wanted to walk crazy distances. Friends are supportive, but lots of people are bemused by my passion for this.'

She joined Wonder Walkers in 2009 and has been a regular contributor to chat forums where she has shared successes and setbacks — and sought support — ever since: 'I get a buzz from all the feedback. Although I'm quite a disciplined and self-contained person, I'm also very communicative and I thrive on the feedback.'

Tanja does walks of up to 10 kilometres and well over that at least three days a week, and has done this consistently for a couple of years. In the 18-month period up to June 2011, she had logged well over an incredible 2000 kilometres, plus five half-marathons, five off-road events and too many 10-kilometre walks to count.

Mostly she walks alone, setting out in all directions from home, often with music or a podcast plugged into just one ear. She says it is essential to have the other ear tuned into what is going on around her in the interests of walking safely, but the podcasts feed her mind, adding interest to the exercise.

Some days she walks 10 kilometres each way to work, leaving home at 5.45am.

It is a solitary exercise regime that she says suits her personality and is good for her wellbeing.

Below is a sample page from Tanja's walk diary:

April 15 – May 2, 2011

May 2 walked 28.2km around the city

April 28 walked 7.5 km

April 25 walked 11km to the park from home and back again

April 24 walked 17km to Panmure Basin, twice around then up Mt Wellington and down again, home and down to Sylvia Park

April 21 walked 10km on a local loop

April 20 walked 6.4km on local errands

April 18 walked 10km Sunrise Walk for Hospice

April 15 walked 10km

Chapter 8

KITTED OUT IN STYLE FOR FUNCTION AND GOOD FORM

One of the best reasons for buying special walking gear is that a girl likes to look good and feel good even when puffing along the neighbourhood pavements. And if you like those tops and pants, you are going to be more likely to want to pull them on and go.

But of course there are other equally good reasons for buying clothing and shoes that are specially developed for regular walking over a reasonable distance and a range of surfaces. Not only will you be comfortable, but you could be preventing injury and damage to yourself. Whatever your budget, you won't regret buying shoes that have been especially designed with the sort of fit, comfort and performance you will need for more than the occasional stroll.

Wherever there is a shopping mall there is likely to be a big sports gear store where you will get a good workout just making your way around the amazing range of stuff, or maybe wondering where to start! With so much to choose from and so much to consider over such a big price range, you will want to start shopping with an idea of what would be most suitable for you. As with most things, you get what you pay for. If budget is an issue, get to know your brands because the sales come around pretty regularly.

Feet first

Feet come in many shapes and sizes but one thing is for sure: if they hurt, you won't be happy, much less walking very far. Your feet can be long, narrow or wide, and the arch of your foot may be high, you may be a bit flat footed with low arches, or somewhere in between. Feet are complex things with an incredible number of bits that need to be in balance to avoid painful and debilitating trouble.

Our arches help us adapt to changing ground underfoot, flexing and distributing weight as we walk. One easy way to get a picture of your foot shape is to simply dip them into water then make a careful footprint on a thick piece of paper. If you are flat-footed you will get a long, full wide image. With higher arches there will almost no imprint from heel to sole.

Choosing shoes for walking

Your walking shoes will arguably have to do much greater service than your party shoes, and getting the right pair for you will help prevent injuries and the development of calluses and blisters.

Walking has less impact on your feet than running. If you like, you can choose running shoes or a cross-trainer type which are lighter-weight and will have more padding and other features, giving more overall comfort and stability, which might appeal for faster walking.

Shoes made especially for walking have cushioning under the ball of the foot. They are likely to look a bit sturdier and heavier than running shoes, and offer various options for arch support. Some walking shoes and their linings are more waterproof than others, giving a range of choice for walking in wet places or hot, dry climates.

Whatever the features, fit is the major consideration and the shoe that fits well is the shoe for you. But before you get down to trying them on in the store, ask which ones might be good for you so you can whittle down the choices to manageable proportions.

And once you know your ideal walking shoes, you will be able to pick up top of the line models in the sporting good sales pretty regularly. The more you walk, the faster you will be wearing out shoes.

Some women hate the heavy and not so flattering look of walking shoes, and are tempted to buy for style rather than function. Women who are serious about getting into walking do not make the same mistake twice.

Steps to great walking shoes
- Know your foot shape.
- Research the shoe range and seek advice.
- Remember: comfort is key.
- Choose for your climate — wet or dry?
- Choose running shoes if you prefer them.
- Replace your shoes as soon as they show signs of wear.

Socks matter

Forget cotton socks: they do not have the right qualities to deal with sweat, keep moisture under control, and keep blisters at bay. Good socks for walking are made from materials known as wicking fabrics. They are specially designed to take moisture away from your skin, and therefore prevent softening and the inevitable formation of painful blisters.

Walking socks will have a little soft padding where you need it — under your heel, the balls of your feet and your toes. For a snug fit they are in the shape of a foot and they will be firm and not bunch up in your shoes.

You pay for design and performance, but the latest in walking socks last for ages.

Walking clothes that perform with style

Ditch the old track pants and baggy tees on the grounds of both function and style. They won't make you feel good, and they can flap and chafe if they are heavy, rigid or bulky. Besides cotton can't perform for repetitive exercise and will soon become soggy and uncomfortable.

Clothes made for walking are smooth and move with you, keeping you warm in winter and absorbing perspiration in hot weather. There are all sorts of synthetic fabric blends to suit all climates. In winter, choose walking tops that you can layer. You start out cosy, but you can peel off layers as you start to warm up. For the layer next to your skin, choose fabrics that will draw away moisture and let out excess body heat to keep you cool and stop you feeling sweaty and clammy. Avoid shorts, and instead choose pants that are smooth, fitted and comfortable.

For wet weather, choose jackets in fabrics that will allow your body to breathe.

Consider adding some reflective spots to your shoes and clothes as a little safety precaution if you will be walking in poorly lit places.

Sporting good stores have clothes that are right for walking in your environment as well as lots that are engineered to perform in different or more extreme conditions. Most stores have some knowledgeable staff, so ask what is right for you.

Hats and visors

Don't forget your head or the need to be insulated and to keep the weather off your face. If you are out walking most days, sun damage is a serious threat to your skin.

Dressing for success

Make sure your walking wardrobe:
- is made from fabrics that breathe and keep moisture off your skin
- contains the right garments for your walking conditions
- has clothes you can layer in winter
- is not made from cotton
- has walking gear you look good in
- features reflective spots for walking in the dark.

PROFILE

Gearing up for a grand and glamorous goal

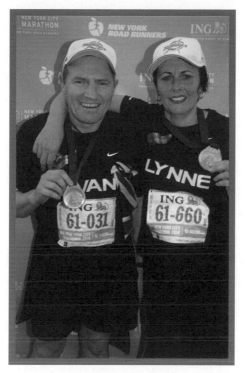

Evan and Lynne Kroll sporting their New York marathon medals.

Back in 2009 the New York Marathon 2010 popped into Lynne Kroll's head quite by chance. It was her answer to an unexpected challenge from someone working out alongside her in her local gym: 'You're here working out all the time — what's your goal?'

At that moment, Lynne, who had always just worked out — and walked — didn't really have a goal. But, hey, why not? And overnight she dared to dream up something far bigger than pounding the streets of her home town, as she had done for years. She would walk the New York Marathon before she turned fifty. Her husband, Evan, took little persuading to sign up for the marathon with her and join her on the training programme.

Forty-nine-year-old Lynne was no stranger to lots and lots of walking, and had been putting in around an hour a day, five days a week for nearly 20 years; as a result of which she had made and sustained a dramatic weight loss. As a young mother she had tipped the scales at around 97 kilograms, and in her own words was 'totally over it. I was tired of myself as a big person.'

Two decades on and the exercise habits of gym and walking every day have kept her around a very much trimmer, fitter and healthier 65 kilograms. Her exercise regime was quite easily stepped up to include big weekend walks with her husband over the hills, and she was confident she would do well in New York. Indeed, Lynne was hoping to better the times she had done in the two national marathons she had completed.

And, despite a painful injury to her foot, she finished in five hours and seven minutes, well under the five and a half hours she and Evan had anticipated. The race day was a fantastic experience, but so too was the huge support from New Yorkers for the event, the fabulous entertainment supporting it, and the friendship run on the preceding day with thousands of competitors running — many in national dress.

'I will never forget the sights, the sounds, the people and the excitement of it all. The city and all the thousands of New Yorkers cheering us on just blew me away.'

Doing the New York marathon, like other marathons anywhere in the world, brings its own set of challenges, and attention to detail pays off, including having the right gear for this great walking challenge. For example, competitors wake and leave by buses for the start line as early as 3am on a freezing winter's morning. Waiting for the race to start is very uncomfortable without rugs and something to rest on.

Wearing gear that shows where you are from is a great way to get support from the crowd when you want a boost, and Lynne says wearing their finisher medals drew very friendly gestures from New Yorkers for days afterwards. Layers of clothing and gloves proved invaluable, too, but they had to be discarded along the way as Lynne warmed up. 'A waste, but my only option was to ditch stuff as I went.'

She says be prepared once you have finished to cope with the frustrations of trying to get away from the finish line along with crowds of others. 'We would have hobbled for half an hour to get back to our gear bags.'

Tips for the New York Marathon

- Be well prepared for the freezing local pre-event conditions.
- Wear clothing that reflects the country you are from.
- Be comfortable.
- Be prepared for big crowds, both before and afterwards.

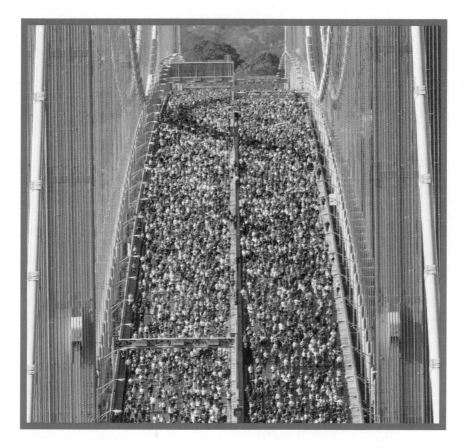

Thousands of marathon competitors foot it over a New York bridge.

Chapter 9

WALKING GROUPS ARE TAKING OFF

There are walking groups for most age groups springing up all over the place. If you are finding it hard to find a regular buddy to go with and you are not keen to be regularly walking alone, joining a group could be the answer.

Being part of a group could be the key to keeping you committed to regular walking for months or years. It could also widen your social circle, give you a ready-made team to join events, or take you much further afield. The strength in numbers brings lots of benefits — even fund-raising opportunities!

Finding a walking group that suits you is really only limited by your imagination and determination to seek out what feels right for you. You could try several before making a choice. The internet makes this research easy, but you could also try local fitness centres and your own workplace, networks you have through your job or other organisations you might belong to, from choirs to parent groups and sports clubs.

You might like to start out with a group of friends and train for a one-off fun walk event if you are not ready for a longer-term commitment. Online communities such as www.wonderwalkers.co.nz are a good place to look for women near you who like to walk. As we have seen already, the women who belong to Wonder Walkers are widely scattered but they chat on line, support each other, and of course share news and tips about all things to do with their common interest in walking, and more. Sometimes they meet up at events.

Starting your own group could be as easy as putting a notice into a community newspaper or community newsletters, or putting up a flyer in community centres, churches, club rooms and medical centres to recruit fellow walkers.

Once you get started you will want a plan to help keep the momentum up and prevent any fall-off in enthusiasm. Look out for fun walks of 5 or 10 kilometres coming up in your region. In most cities and sizeable towns there will be quite a few you could work up to doing every year. Maybe a weight loss challenge could also be another motivator for your group.

It is a good idea to have a meeting to start off with, where you can sort out things such as how far you want to walk and how often, and the visions you share for this group. Having sufficient numbers to split into at least two groups — one for brisk to average walkers, and another slower group — would be likely to widen the appeal of your group to walkers of differing fitness.

Set up email contacts and telephone numbers so you can easily keep in touch — and keep everyone committed. No doubt each member will come up with good walking routes and a coffee stop to finish up at.

These are some details you could sort out to increase your chances of making it a sustainable group.

• Is it about fitness, fun, weight loss, support, or training?
• How often and on what days will you walk?
• Morning, evening or weekend walks, or a mix of all?
• How far will you go and how fast?
• Is it feasible to split into groups of varying fitness levels?
• What will you do in bad weather?
• Will your group enter events?
• Who will be your co-ordinator?
• How big do you want your group to grow?
• Is the group a long-term prospect?

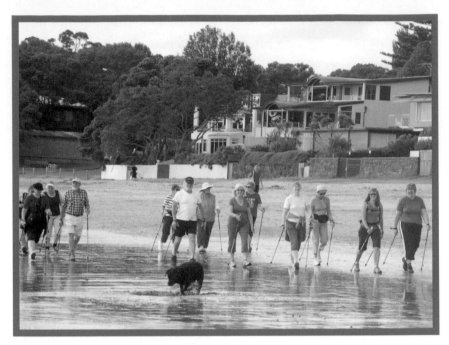

Why not take the dog as well?

PROFILE

Online walking buddies

The answer to finding regular walking buddies for one 55-year-old, Elaine, was to join the online community of women on www.wonderwalkers.co.nz.

When she first started walking regularly, her dog Maggie was her usual companion, but now the aging family pet can't keep up. Nevertheless, Elaine says she is very happy walking alone, spurred on by the walking buddies she connects with online. As 'WWElaine' she regularly dips in and out of the website chat forum, reporting on progress, or the lack of it, and her resolve to keep going.

'I'm not a group walker, but I enjoy the connection with this group and the feedback. It has been very valuable to keeping up motivation. When I am good, I am very good; and when I am bad, I'm no good at all. And the girls hear about it,' says Elaine. Since she joined the forum in July 2008, around 200 posts have popped up from WWElaine sharing titbits on her progress over three years and exchanging snatches of news and encouragement with other regular contributors all over the country.

She says she walks for both mind and weight loss, adding that she still has a couple of kilograms she would like to shed. With a busy full-time job, she has to get out on foot early in the morning before starting her working day.

'Walking for me is a discipline, but one that makes the effort so worthwhile. I read once that walking early in the day, before breakfast, speeds the metabolism for the whole day ahead. I made the effort to do this; however, the benefits are so much more than what it does for my metabolism. For me it is thinking time, a time for planning my day, and I find that everything goes so much better for me — I have sharper thinking and more motivation to do household chores. I also enjoy relaxing walks after work on the beach or around the area I live in. Walking is one of Nature's best kept secrets.'

This is a little peek at WWElaine's online walk diary from April 2011 when she was resolving to get back into her routine. Having this simple diary of her walking on line is one of the things she loves about being part of the website community and the exchange of friendly talk-oriented banter she can go in search of at the stroke of a key.

April 10, walked 4.5km. Back on track and trying hard.

April 11, walked 4.5km. Sunday to beach, market, shopping etc.

April13, walked 3.5km. Started back daily early mornings. From home to beach and back then out again with Maggie for a quick 10 minutes after.

April 14, walked 2.5km. With Maggie to school and back — she coped well. Considering I've not done this for ages this will be the balance for me and her in the mornings. We will do longer at weekends.

April 15, walked 2.5km. To school and back on more challenging route. Maggie okay but v tired when we got home.

April 18, walked 8.5km. Around local beaches then slowed down, a bit of a browse around market and coffee with Mag. Speeded up for uphill home, the long way round. Felt great.

April 20, walked 2.9km. To Mobil garage, took 27 minutes but not as far as I planned. Try again tomorrow night.

April 21, walked 2.00km. Early morning to school and back with Mags, Planning to try for further tonight and will leave earlier. Good start today. At desk at 8 and currently eating my breakfast cereal!

PROFILE

Devonport Y's Walkers:
going strong for a quarter century

Fitness, friendship, picnics, parties, hip operations, funerals, romances and much more! It's all there in the 25-year story of the now quite senior group of walkers who make up the Devonport Walking Group. A redoubtable bunch of up to 40 women (and men) who head out on foot together around their beautiful historic seaside suburb on a number of weekday mornings.

This urban walking group is thought to be the longest running in New Zealand, and with a fair smattering of its original members still in the ranks, the ages of many have crept up into late 70s and beyond. It is estimated that over 200 people, plus overseas visitors, have walked with this group at some time, but for years there has been a large core of regulars. They have walks scheduled three mornings a week, but not everyone makes it that often. Age aside, it is not just a stroll with this lot: walks cover up to seven kilometres over an hour or so.

The group was started 25 years ago by Pat McKay and her husband, Jim, and the couple have run it ever since. Pat saw the potential appeal for a group like this in her neighbourhood after discovering the Y's walking concept when it was introduced elsewhere in the city. Then in her mid-50s, she put together a flyer and delivered it around the village, not forgetting the waiting rooms of local doctors. Just five people turned up for the first walk.

'That was a good start and I was determined to make it work. Why walk on your own, I thought, when a group could be a lot of fun for a lot of people.'

Currently there are 80 paid-up members. Many joined in midlife, but, although the majority are now well into their senior years, younger people frequently join them.

'It has been very, very successful, and I know a lot of people would attribute their good health in later life to walking with us on a regular basis. We've often had new members who have been sent along by local doctors.'

'It is a great way to make friends, have a good social life and to look out for each other as we're all getting older.'

But there have been many other spinoffs besides fitness. At the end of each walk this healthy looking bunch fill up a local café and spill out in a jolly babble onto the pavement before going their separate ways. The social benefits do not stop there, though. They have regular dinners together, and parties where members bring a plate and a bottle of wine to celebrate those big birthdays with a zero in them. Mid-winter lunches, picnics and cricket games are on the calendar, too. Members swap books and recipes.

They are a strong support network for each other in sickness or in crisis times, and some, who are now partners, found romance late in life through joining the walkers.

The Devonport Walkers are very much part of their local landscape and no longer need any promotion as a vibrant community group. Members pay just $10 a year, a portion of which goes to Hospice and to the local community house. Everyone is asked to work out new routes to add a bit of variety, and everyone finds their own pace, with the fast pack out front, the big bunch in the middle and those who regularly tail at the back.

The seaside town is the sort of place many settle in and stay forever, so there is a very strong community spirit which has probably contributed both to the longevity and the success of this walking group. Nevertheless it is a story that could easily be replicated in many other towns as well.

'Devonport is a beautiful place to walk, but any community could have a group like this if people believe in the benefits and are keen enough to make it happen,' says Pat. 'Like us, they'd soon get to enjoy it and be so much better off for it.'

Chapter 10

BABY TAKE A WALK IN THE PARK: WALKING WITH BABIES, TODDLERS AND BIGGER KIDS

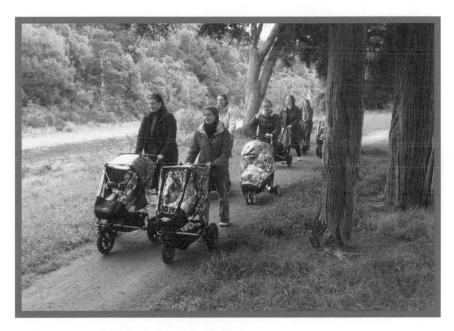

Mothers walk together with their babies.

There is nothing new about popping a baby in a pram — or a toddler in a pushchair — and taking a stroll together. Never mind the exercise you will be getting, the universal need to just get out of the house for a while propels mothers everywhere, whatever the weather.

Generations of new mothers have accepted some of the seemingly inevitable downside that comes with the joy of having a child: losing their figures and their fitness, losing a bit of confidence, social isolation and loneliness, fatigue and maybe even postnatal depression. The new generation doesn't have to accept those things sitting down, because health professionals, research scientists, community organisations and kindred spirits are pulling together, urging them to make social contact and an exercise date a real option.

These days women are mobilising to make more of walking with little ones, and they are getting together to wheel their infants in groups in a growing trend dubbed 'pram-walking' or 'buggy-walking'. And whether it is just a couple of women or a whole fleet wheeling along together, these walking groups are a great option for mothers and babies.

There are lots of benefits to joining one of these groups. You can lose weight, meet new people, tone up a little, have fun and boost your mood. It is virtually free and is a regular motivation to get out with other young mothers. With small children to work around, it is never easy finding time to exercise, so pram- or buggy-walking is a great way to actively take care of yourself and socialise without the hassle of finding child care. What's more, it is a firm date to look forward to at a time of life when going out anywhere is much more difficult than it used to be. While arrangements with friends can easily fall over, your buggy-walk day could be a sure thing.

For so many mothers who are tired, a bit lonely, a bit blue and finding it hard to get enough exercise or just fit in a bit of 'me time', pram-walking ticks lots of boxes for overall wellbeing. And like walking in general, it has the seal of approval from health researchers. A study in Australia found that a 12-week programme improved the fitness and reduced the symptoms of postnatal depression of the women in the group — hardly surprising really.

Where are the pram-walkers?

If you live in a bigger city you may be able to find a pram or buggy walking group to join. Some towns and cities in Australia and New Zealand have annual or more regular events where you could give it a try and make contact with others who in your region who might like to make up a regular walking group. These groups are springing up in Australia and the UK, many with the backing of local councils and health institutions. Many can be found with a quick search of the internet, with the sort of detail that could be useful to others starting out together. Of course, many smaller groups are just getting out there without formal support in the shape of funding, leadership or promotion. They're just doing it!

The Wellington Buggy Walkers

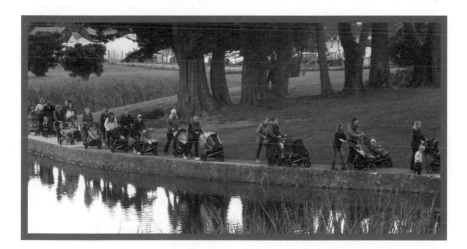

Buggy-walking with friends in pleasant surroundings can be reinvigorating.

Young Wellington mothers are lucky enough to have buggy-walks very well organised for them. The buggy-walking programme in New Zealand's capital city has gathered great momentum since 2006, when it was launched.

The organisers have put a bit of work into checking out all the walks in advance, and they post details of the upcoming events on the website www.buggywalk.co.nz. Most routes are off-road, and for many mothers exploring their city's rugged but beautiful outdoors and discovering great spots for return visits has been an extra bonus to joining this adventurous group. They have found there is great strength in numbers when it comes to getting out there with littlies in tow.

In good weather the walkers tackle buggy-friendly tracks in parks and forests around the region. In winter, well wrapped up for the elements, this big group of mothers and infants mobilise on more urban routes. There is a leader for the walks, which are suitable for all ages and abilities and take about an hour.

On the first Thursday morning of every month upwards of 150 women turn out with their kids in buggies, and some are joined by grandparents, too. There's a Facebook page to support the group where members join discussions, post lots of photos from their expeditions together, and generally contribute to this vibrant community of walkers. They make new friends and get all the fun and benefits on offer from being part of an active group.

At Sport Wellington the co-ordinator Rachel Spriggens says the buggy-walking programme is now very well established with nearly 300 members. The women and children come from all over the city, and Rachel says social media, including their Facebook page, have played a big part in both promoting the venture and providing a communications and networking system. Women at home with their kids are now so much easier to engage with and motivate than they were even a decade ago, thanks to the wizardry of IT.

The buggy-walking programme has been such a success that smaller groups have sprung up in a number of Wellington suburbs. Some antenatal coffee groups use the chance to join up with these organised outings to enjoy their regular meetings on foot, rather than gather together to eat, drink and swap stories in each other's living rooms.

The faces change slowly over time as kids outgrow their buggies, and Rachel Spriggens says putting energy into recruiting membership is an important part of keeping this programme viable and active for years to come.

Five years on, the foundation babies are at school and their mothers may have moved on to new things, but the Wellington Buggy Walkers keep on keeping on. Once a year they make a startling and happy sight when as many as 800 converge for an annual buggy walk around the pathways of the city's beautiful Botanic Gardens.

Getting rolling

Setting up a successful, sustainable pram- or buggy-walking group — from a small group of local mothers, to a larger ongoing local programme — takes a bit of hard work and organisation to make it happen and to keep it rolling.

In the Australian city of Darebin, determined women made it happen by getting their city council on board to set up the Darebin Pram Walkers programme and to provide the backup that would see it take off and thrive.

The Darebin City Pram Walkers

The Darebin Pram Walkers Committee was set up by the local city council. The committee members knew a lot about the health and wellbeing of mothers and children, they had administrative support, they had the blessing of the city and they had funding.

They were able to pay a co-ordinator to run the pram-walking group and they found this job was very important to the success of a group that is proving to be a lifeline and great friend to young mothers in the city.

They also had the means to produce an attractive and useful guide for setting up a pram-walking programme, Baby Take a Walk in the Park, as a resource to share with other councils, parents and communities to start their own local groups.

'This guide aims to make accessible to others what has been learnt by trial and error, to ensure that programmes are developed within a relatively short time frame, and more importantly, that they survive to provide a much needed and beneficial support to new parents,' says the introduction.

Aware of the multicultural makeup of their city, they included an introduction to their guide in a number of languages, including Italian, Greek, Chinese, Arabic, Macedonian and Vietnamese.

The path for Darebin Pram Walkers mothers was not always smooth or straight, though, and the shaky start could have been the end of this new idea when it was first mooted a decade ago — well before it became a great opportunity for young mothers all over the region. Now it's probably the longest-running group of its kind in the world.

When a group of nurses launched the group at a local park in September 2001, there was a promising turnout of 50 mums with prams and babies. Six walks were chosen, and they were led by volunteers from among the parents. Alas, by January 2002 there was only one walk remaining. Undeterred, that little band of nurses and mothers went looking for the backing that would take this wobbly pilot project to a community programme. Countless women love them for it.

The women behind the success of the Darebin Pram Walkers soon realised there were quite a few things to consider and a number of key ingredients in making this particular group for the mothers of quite young babies popular and successful.

For example, they knew that these women were likely to be the new parents of young babies. They could be sleep-deprived, still recovering physically from the birth, not very confident about caring for their baby, possibly without much social support or battling depression, and maybe nervous about joining a new group.

All round, many were likely be at quite a vulnerable time in their lives, and, in order to provide the potential benefits of this fledgling walk group, the participants would need to be carefully lured in — and nurtured. It was important, therefore, that the walk leader handle them with care and be welcoming and encouraging.

These are snippets of feedback from mothers with young babies who joined up: 'I had a difficult pregnancy, which meant I had done little exercise during the pregnancy. It was wonderful to go on an invigorating walk with others and get my strength and fitness back,' said one mother.

Another said: 'The really big benefits were that it got me out of the house and doing something healthy with my bub that didn't cost money. It didn't matter if bub cried. Getting out and not being alone were the most important things. The group was really friendly and supportive.'

The organisers drew up a list of the key lessons they learned and suggestions for setting up a group.

Tips from the Darebin Pram Walkers for running a successful group

• A dedicated co-ordinator is essential.
• While new parents have many things in common, they come from a diverse range of backgrounds and situations — this should be considered when setting up a programme so that all new parents have an opportunity to participate.
• Parents are a transitional group — promotion needs to be constant to fill the ranks.
• A funding source will be needed.
• Programme partners are extremely valuable for their knowledge, expertise and encouragement.
• Volunteer walk leaders are an important force in the programme.
• The support of others in the community who work with mothers and babies can be a big help in recruiting walkers.
• Parklands and open areas are more suitable for walking groups with prams.
• Having a coffee stop en route increases participation and gives people more of a chance to chat to others.
• A launch or regular special events will make the group or programme more popular.

Get rolling along together

If you are keen to start a group you will want to think about whether it is feasible in your area and how big you want it to be. Would you want it to be just a group for your own pram- and buggy-pushing years, or something that rolls on for others in years to come? Who would join up and how would they find out about it? Would someone in your business community print flyers for you? Could you get the local paper to help you spread the word? Could you get listed on local websites?

Walking routes

• Is it suitable terrain for prams and buggies?
• How long is the round trip?
• Can you walk two abreast, chatting as you walk?
• Does it cross over busy roads?
• Is there shelter or shade at least part of the way?
• Are there toilets along the route?
• Can you build in a coffee stop or rest stop along the way?

Pram-walking for babies

A happier, healthier mother has to be good for babies, but there are some things to check before popping a baby in a pram or buggy and taking it out for a walk. While mothers will soon warm up from walking, the infant won't be getting the benefits of that warm-up and will be much more vulnerable to the effects of the elements — and to the impact of dodgy terrain. So make sure the baby is well protected from the weather and suitably dressed, and take plenty of water for both of you.

Also, consider the following points:
• Can you find shade and a place to take a break?
• Will you need to stop for breastfeeding on the way?
• Will your baby be safe and comfortable at all times?
• What will you do with your baby if you stop for coffee?
• Can you make a nappy change?
• Is the walk too long?
• Is your pram or buggy up to the task?

Take care of those muscles

You may be a little out of shape after having a child, and carrying kids and pushing prams bring extra stresses. Make sure you are in good time to take part in the warm-up and stretches before you set off and when you finish — the next day you will be glad you did!

For all walkers, stretching your leg muscles is important for preventing injury and soreness. But pushing a pram can make your shoulders, upper back and neck tight, too, so it is wise to pay attention to stretching these areas also.

Adjust the height of the pram or buggy handle if you can, to avoid stooping as you walk with it.

Walking with bigger kids

Walking is also very good for children, particularly if you are concerned that they are inactive or in danger of being overweight. But since they are unlikely to be lured along by the promise of scenery or health benefits at a tender age, getting them started may not be so easy.

Motivating kids to walk will be much more likely with a bit of planning and ingenuity, combined with a very positive and patient approach. No doubt, some will take to it more readily than others, particularly in families with a more outdoors and active lifestyle. But even if your kids are largely couch potatoes and a bit resistant to exercise, it can be done.

Not only is it good for them and a great habit to instil for a lifetime, it is also great for mothers who like to walk and welcome ways to alleviate the dreaded scenario of coping with bored offspring. And it is also a cheap outing in the school holidays.

If you want children to get out walking regularly, you will have to work a bit to make it sound like fun, or at least more interesting than staying home. You could go it alone, but doing it with friends and other mothers and their children is likely to make for a much jollier outing. There can be strength in numbers when it comes to occupying kids.

Work out a plan according to the age and ability of the walkers, the weather, and the environment. Obvious choices are a beach ramble or nature trails with plenty of points of interest. Add interest by collecting things as you go (unless it is a 'look but don't take' zone). Maybe you could make it a bit competitive, with the small walkers drawing what they saw or writing a story about it when they get back home. Or just take photographs for a creative dimension.

If attention spans are short, or boredom threatens, try the good old 'eye spy' routine with the added challenge of spotting a number of objects that are the same colour or start with the same letter. Perhaps you could add in a few treats and rewards, too, ensuring a little more enthusiasm. Let them take along their own little pack with water and a snack.

Older children might be motivated if part of the purpose is to collect litter, deliver flyers, or to reach an interesting destination holding the promise of more excitement and enjoyment, such as a park, an ice cream shop, a local attraction.

The prospect of a treasure hunt at the final destination will urge them along. So, too, would a post-walk get-together for a shared lunch back home with their walking friends or a picnic outdoors.

A bit of advance promotion would help to talk up the walk before you attempt your first foray. How you make it happen is limited only by your imagination and determination. Other mothers will love you for it, and your kids might have such a good time that they'll want to go out walking again and again.

Once you have put walking on to the family schedule and have a few kilometres successfully covered without too many complaints, consider planning something more ambitious for them to tackle. There are many family- and child-friendly 5-kilometre fun walks in most places that primary schoolchildren could do and enjoy with a bit of preparation.

Tips for walking with kids

• Make a plan.

• Make it fun.

• Make sure they have suitable shoes and clothing to be comfortable.

• Get other mothers to join you.

• Include some incentives and rewards.

• Look out for child-friendly walking events.

PROFILE

A pram-walking group was a lifesaver

Emma Darragh-Heath writes:

My two sons and I recently hiked for five hours up The Pinnacles in the stunning Kauaeranga Valley. Breathlessly scaling hundreds of steps, ladders and handholds in rocks, we finally made it! It was a proud victory for all of us and good confirmation that I was on the 'right track' as a mum.

Looking back eight years ago to my first-born's first year, I am very grateful for circumstances which led us to a love of walking in the great outdoors.

Back in 2000, the hospitality industry lured my husband and me to Melbourne. Two years down the track we were in a little semi-detached house in suburbia with a small, constantly crying baby. If there was a list of factors that could trigger postnatal depression, I suspect I may have had just about all of them:

• colicky unsettled baby who wouldn't sleep

• husband working night shifts

• living far away from family

• young mother, no experience with babies

• not knowing anyone in my community

• not knowing any other mothers

• no job for the first time ever

• a newborn baby in the wet cold winter.

Simply getting through each day became an arduous task, interspersed with moments of utter despair. My baby son's screams echoed against the walls of the small house.

In desperation, I began to go out walking him in his pram every day. I was exhausted and every step was excruciating and tiresome, as I realised how physically tired I was. My baby boy screamed with my every step. But then, after a while there would be silence. The motion soothed him, and he settled to a long, deep sleep. I began to sense the warmth of the sun on my skin, and the rhythm of movement.

It felt good! I became aware of my surroundings and each walk became a new adventure. I soon discovered a labyrinth of parks and grassy paths in a city I had not previously taken the time to get to know beyond its restaurants, bars and boutiques.

An advertisement in the local newspaper piqued my interest in walking with a group. The local council had initiated neighbourhood pram-walkers' groups, where mums and babies could meet at a designated place for twice-weekly walks in the local area. I didn't know anyone in my suburb and, as I was quite young and didn't have any existing friends who were mothers, I thought it would be a good opportunity to meet other women who were first-time mothers.

I was nervous as I walked down my street to the arranged meeting spot. I needn't have been. There were 12 of us that first day, and within minutes we were chatting like old friends. We walked two-by-two along the Darebin Creek, and stopped for a coffee break at an outdoor café. Then we walked back, refreshed, revitalised and ready to face another round of night-feeds, nappies and not much sleep.

The pram-walkers' group shaped a new chapter of my life as a mother. I had somewhere I had to be, twice a week at a fixed time. It was important to me, so I made it happen every time, on time. This was significant, as I felt I had turned my whole life upside down trying to accommodate the demands of an unsettled newborn. He came first in every other way, but this was a twice-weekly date where I made my own wellbeing a priority. I didn't miss a walk — rain, hail or shine. It was important.

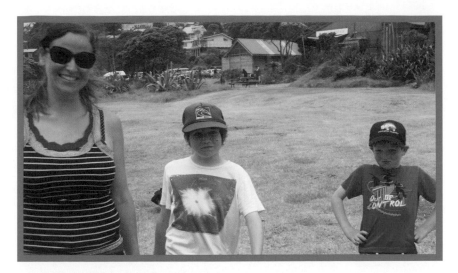

Emma Darragh-Heath with her sons.

I had also attended new mothers' coffee mornings organised by the local health centre. I often left those mornings feeling lonely and inadequate as all the conversation centred on the babies and I seemed to be the only one having a hard time.

In sharp contrast, talking with pram-walking mothers was an honest, heart-warming experience. Often we didn't even talk babies (unheard of at the coffee groups)! The fresh air and tranquillity of Nature made for a relaxed, easy atmosphere. We felt safe to vent our frustrations and be supported in our tiny victories. True friendships were forged with all those footsteps.

It is only with the benefit of hindsight that I can fully appreciate the positive impact that the pram-walkers' group had on me and on my family. I kept walking with the same core group of women for a whole year, before leaving the area. Those women became incredibly supportive friends, our children became friends, and our husbands also became friends.

Some of the women had lived in the neighbourhood for several years, and it wasn't until they became pram walkers that they got to know each other. In that group a very real sense of community and belonging was fostered at a time when its members were particularly vulnerable.

I will always be grateful for those people behind the initiative of the Darebin Pram Walkers' Group. In friendship and in fitness, I regained a sense of self and a spirit of purpose and positivity. Without walking, I look back and see that I was on a slippery slope down the path of postnatal depression. The pram-walkers' group set me on a different course and showed me the tremendous power of a simple daily walk. I share that with my beautiful growing boys today, and they too conquer the seemingly insurmountable. Walking makes all of us happy.

Chapter 11

MALL-WALKERS: GETTING ACTIVE IN THE HOTTEST AND COLDEST OF CLIMATES

Many mall-walkers are old enough to be the mothers or grandmothers of the new generation of pram-walkers, but they have one thing in common: they want to get out walking on a regular basis and they have found a way to make sure they do just that.

Mall-walking is another relatively new thing in the worldwide walking picture. For a decade or more, whether it is windy or wet, freezing cold or unbearably hot, determined walkers have been heading off to malls and joining big bands of buddies on a couple of mornings a week.

No one knows where mall-walking really first began, but once the idea of early morning walking in shopping centres was put into words, the term 'mall-walking' came into being and a new trend came to life. It has caught on fast in a number of countries, particularly those with extreme climates, as a sure way to keep up a regular walking schedule.

The many benefits are obvious. Shopping malls offer a safe, controlled environment in all climates, at all times of the year. They are mostly flat, the ground is even and unlikely to throw up any obstacles. And in cities, many are more than large enough to provide a walk of 45 minutes or more from a couple of circuits, and you won't have to share the walk with dogs, kids, cyclists or other hazards that can and do trip up some walkers in the great outdoors. If you tire, you can pause for a bit of window shopping or easily find a place to sit and rest, or even have a coffee.

In mild climates, regular mall-walking women are usually a greying bunch and often grannies who are committed to their indoor walking routine. But wherever freezing days or blistering heat make the outdoors less than hospitable, mall-walkers can be all ages, all shapes and sizes, and at many different levels of fitness.

Many of the successful groups that have sustained themselves and grown their ranks have a leader who sets the pace and makes sure that nattering and straggling don't overshadow the core purpose of the group, which is to get sufficient regular exercise to be beneficial to them. Walks start with the warm-up and stretch exercises that are so vital to protecting aging bodies from strain and pain. Typically, they will be on foot for up to an hour before warming down and sitting down for a coffee break together at a café in the mall that will welcome this early morning business from quite a large group.

In 2009, the launch of a mall-walking group in sultry Dubai made it onto international television news. Although in places like the United States and Canada, mall-walkers are quite a common sight, the Dubai group was something new in that part of the world. The group was established to walk in the plush Mall of Emirates five mornings a week. In a place where heat and humidity forces people indoors, it is hardly surprising that local ex-pat women grabbed the chance to get together to exercise in the mall. Some say it has been a lifesaver for them; others say it was great to be on the spot when the shop doors opened at sale time.

In Canada, it is not the heat but the freezing winter that keeps people inside, and taking a walk with a group in the cosy and pleasant environment of a mall outside of shopping hours is something people of all ages do there. On their website, the Health Foundation of Canada promotes mall-walking for maintaining cardiovascular health. The foundation says studies have shown that walking two and a half hours per week (30 minutes, 5 days per week) cuts the risk of developing cardiovascular and coronary heart diseases by 50 per cent. They are working to spread the word on the benefits, and list eight mall-walker progammes to choose from across Toronto and the surrounding region.

In the United States — the land of the giant shopping complex — some call it 'mallercise', and there has been a big increase in participation and programmes on offer. The majority are older citizens, and, although they have found a new formula for fun and fitness, some say walking in the tempting environment of shop windows is making their wallets a bit thinner, too.

The British latched on to this trend once they had spotted it in the United States, and although their malls may be puny things by comparison, the movement is slowly building up. They certainly have the right weather for it!

British media could not really decide whether walking in malls for exercise was a bit daft or a great idea, but they were curious nevertheless. This is an excerpt from an article by Anthony Gardner in the UK newspaper *The Daily Telegraph* on 8 July 2009:

> House of Fraser, John Lewis, Marks & Spencer: these are the main compass points for walkers at Bluewater. The shopping centre in Kent may be enormous, but once you have a fix on its three corners, your chances of getting lost are minimal, even if a thick fog should steal in from the coast. Those of us who struggle to read maps need never trouble the emergency services again.
>
> Easy orientation and protection from the elements are two obvious advantages of mall walking. There are no treacherous surfaces, unless someone has spilt their cappuccino outside Starbucks.
>
> If you feel faint, you can sit down and order a full English breakfast at Café Zest; if you want to go to the loo, the on-site facilities are infinitely preferable to a thorny copse. There may not be anything in the way of scenery, but for some the windows of Tommy Hilfiger will do.
>
> If 'mallercise' is still a novelty in Britain, it is because we have only a handful of venues large enough to provide a reasonable circuit.

Almost all the takers are women, partly, the leader believes, because chatting and window shopping play an important part: 'I think women like to socialise more, whereas men tend to say, "Let's go to the gym and be done with it." A lot of our ladies come in pairs.'

Take Lisa Tyler, who has driven 30 miles from Hertfordshire to meet up with her friend Susie Rizzo: 'We're both pretty fit,' she says. 'I went to the Brecon Beacons a few weeks ago to do walking there, and I go to the Cotswolds for long weekends. This has been brilliant — it's a good reason to get up and do something on a Sunday morning.'

It has clearly become a worldwide phenomenon in the 21st century.

How mall-walking groups work

Mostly, the shopping malls initiate mall-walking groups and provide a walk leader, usually someone from a fitness centre. Where local health centres and doctors have given support, some malls organise occasional events, health checks and some discounts for the group members.

Smart mall managements have realised the value of offering this opportunity to their local communities with the goodwill and extra custom it can bring at opening time.

Typically, mall walks start from around 7.15am and finish at about 8.00am, in time for coffee and well ahead of the daily bustle of staff and shoppers. In that time the typical mall-walker takes about 5000 steps. Many are organised in groups of slow, moderate and fast walkers, and should be including warm up and stretch routine. The way any group works will differ from one mall to another, but the idea is still the same.

Many a mall-walking group has given rise to other benefits for the active seniors and women who join them. The typical spinoffs are meeting new people and the opportunity to extend the support networks that can make such a difference to quality of life and all-round enhanced wellbeing for

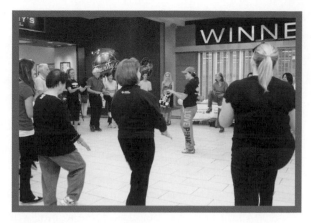

Warming up before they walk. Bayshore Mall, Ottawa. *Photo Amy Symes.*

so many of these walkers who are aging and living alone.

They find strength in numbers, and they often form book clubs or knitting circles, and take the chance to join trips further afield than the shopping centre. While they may never be marathoners, they get many of the same benefits of walkers half their age: exercise, camaraderie, and a great reason to get out of their homes on a regular basis.

If there isn't a group at your mall think about approaching the management to get one started.

Benefits

Mall-walking:
- is good for your health
- provides a regular walking schedule
- is safe
- is predictable
- takes place in a controlled environment
- is sociable
- provides an easy walking surface
- means bathrooms and water are always nearby
- provides a potential network for finding other enjoyable activities.

PROFILE

Elsie Wong — intrepid senior mall-walker

In her 80s, Elsie Wong is currently the oldest member of the large group that strides off around her large local mall two mornings a week, before it opens to the daily throng of shoppers.

Elsie's busy life is packed with a variety of interests and sounds like the schedule of a woman half her age, but Elsie came to mall-walking only a few years ago when a shoulder injury forced her to finally put down her badminton racket.

Not surprisingly, the injury that drove this extraordinarily fit and active woman into the ranks of mall-walkers resulted from a rush of high spirits on Elsie's part and a tree-climbing adventure. 'I fell out of a mandarin tree and went down on my shoulder,' she recalls, as though being up trees was a regular thing for her. 'I saw the last of the fruit at the top and thought I'd go after them before the birds did. I stepped on a rotten branch and down I came. Oh boy, did it hurt. I knew I had done myself a mischief.'

While clearly she could carry on with her regular tap-dancing and community work, the bad shoulder put an end to playing badminton. Happily she spotted a newspaper story about the new mall-walking group starting at the shopping mall and she liked the sound of it.

A foundation member of this mall group, Elsie walks with them two mornings a week for 45 minutes before the group stops for coffee together and then disperses. That is not quite enough walking for her, though, and early on many Saturday mornings she joins an offshoot group of the mall-walkers to do a circuit of the nearby lagoon. Like the others who have met through the walking group, she will often meet up for a get-together or to be part of some other activity.

Elsie says the benefits for her have been friendship, health and fitness. Like some other women who have started walking seriously in later life, she too has trained for and walked half-marathons.

'Without a doubt I am fitter, healthier and stronger than I otherwise might have been at my age, and these are very important benefits to me. It has really strengthened my legs, for example. But it has been wonderful for making new friends and opening up other chances to go out and do things.'

This walking group has a book club, too, and from time to time they organise trips to movies and theatre.

'I might be one of the older ones, and it might seem a bit late in life for all this activity, but I love it. I grew up in the Chinese community and we were brought up working so hard in market gardens that we had no time for leisure. Now it is my time.

'Mall-walking is a wonderful idea. We're mostly a group of retired people and it suits us perfectly. It's safe and dry and you look forward to seeing everyone. It's wonderful for making new friends. It's also a great option for getting older women to make a commitment to getting exercise and keeping fit. All they have to do is put their shoes on and get to the mall.

'I always take the chance to tell people about this and I am just so pleased I heard about it and was lucky enough to be living near enough to take full advantage of this. I really hope so see lots more publicity about mall-walking. At my age, exercise and activity are still a very important part of being happy and well, but none of us might have thought of walking groups in shopping centres until we heard about it.'

Chapter 12

NORDIC WALKING: A BRILLIANT BOOST FROM WALKING POLES

Walking with poles or sticks is far from new. For centuries walkers have carried walking sticks to help them on their travels, whether they were merely headed for the corner store or taking a hike in the country.

In recent years Nordic walking, which employs a specially designed set of poles, has become very popular as a new approach to boosting the many benefits of walking.

Nordic walkers use a pair of poles and a specific technique to enhance the way they walk. And while it may look like a strange way to get around on first sight, walkers all over the world have fast caught on to the benefits of Nordic walking and they are striding out in their millions, hooked on this new sport.

As its name would suggest, the Nordic walking movement started in Finland. Cross-country skiers worked out that they could keep fit through the summer months by still using a pair of poles to help propel them across country on foot. A new sport was born and launched in the late 1990s once a Finnish manufacturer produced the first specially designed walking poles.

Since then, scientific studies have indicated a wide range of health benefits the use of poles can add to regular walking. These range from increased cardiovascular activity to an overall improvement in vitality, with very little extra effort required from the walker.

While the benefits of Nordic walking are still being keenly explored, many health professionals recognise it as an excellent tool for easing and preventing lower back pain and they're recommending it to clients as a workout. The thinking is that the stability provided by the poles enables much great mobility and activates back muscles that might otherwise not get much of a workout.

Within a decade it is estimated more than 8 million people around the world have taken up Nordic walking. In most countries it is now possible to find a qualified instructor and classes where you can quickly learn the technique that will start you off in this style of walking.

What is Nordic walking?

By adding poles to walking you can get a full body workout, take the weight off joints, and greatly enhance the benefits of regular walking by taking you further, faster and working all of your body harder. Walking with the poles combines regular walking with working the muscles in the upper body by adding arm, shoulder and trunk movement as you work with the poles. It also takes the load and wear and tear off your legs and joints.

Nordic walking is an easy way to build up your fitness, regardless of age or health. You can do it at whatever level you like, depending on what you want to get out of it. You will gain immediate benefits from your 30-minute, low-impact walk, but it is likely you will soon be working those poles harder to walk further and tackle more challenging terrain. Walking on sand, for example, is much harder work.

For many fans it has given them the tools and confidence to get back into regular exercise where illness and injury or lack of fitness may have made walking without their trusty poles seem too daunting.

You can go Nordic walking in most places anyone else would like to walk, from parks and beaches to city footpaths. The poles come with little detachable paws for walking on hard pavements.

Benefits

Nordic walking:

• burns more calories than walking with no poles

• engages about 90 per cent of the body's muscle

• takes the weight off your joints

• releases pain and tension around the neck and shoulders

• strengthens the back muscles and increase mobility of spine

• improves co-ordination and balance

• enables you to walk for longer periods

• increases your stability with the support of the poles

• improves posture

• is fun

• can be learned by most people at any age.

How to do it

The technique is relatively easy and quick to learn, but experts say some basic instruction will set you off on the right path to make the most of your new walking poles and to avoid possible injury and disappointment. Although it is not quite as easy as it looks, most people get the hang of it within a few weeks of starting, but the better your technique the more benefits you get from this style of walking. Trying to teach yourself is not recommended.

As you walk, you plant each pole in time with your steps, with the poles pointing diagonally behind you and your arm in time with the opposite leg. Swinging arms and legs alternately, you plant the right pole as your left foot touches the ground and then the left pole is planted as you right foot touches down. You are looking straight ahead with your shoulders relaxed and down, and your upper body leaning slightly forward in a straight line up from your ankle to head. As you master the style you will feel your upper body working and the poles helping to propel you along.

Once you are happily whizzing along on the flat, you can explore using the poles to support you going uphill and downhill, keeping steady and protecting your joints.

Leading the way

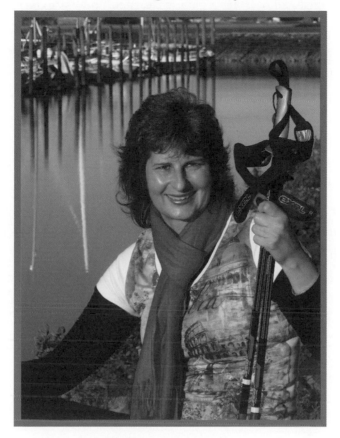

June Stevenson, Nordic walking coach.

June Stevenson is a well-known Nordic walking coach. Becoming an instant convert the moment she tried it, she has been a pioneer in the sport.

'Sport and fitness had always been a big part of my life, but this is just pure magic,' says June with the typical passion and commitment she has put into spreading the bug.

She certainly had the history and the experience to take on another challenge in sport and become a tireless advocate for it. She has had more than 20 years in the health and fitness industry, both as a teacher and a participant. She's been a top basketballer, a runner of marathons, a cyclist, an exercise instructor, and a yoga instructor. Motivator is on the list, too.

Many people are grateful that the magic stuck with her. June runs regular courses all over her region for learners and has to be credited for attracting many into the sport and for building the ranks of the many other instructors now operating around the country, through her commitment to training and certifying according to international standards.

'Once you put the poles into someone's hands it affects their co-ordination. It can be two things too many. But people get into the technique quite quickly and then they are away,' says June.

'I love to teach people how to do it. It just gives me the greatest buzz. I see people attracted to this all the time who couldn't do any other activity. Many are broken-down runners and walkers whose upper body posture has deteriorated, and they comment on the great benefits using poles has for them.'

'Nordic walking is fun, sociable, and very accessible to women of all ages and all levels of fitness. I have had the enjoyment of watching people I've taught take it up with great enthusiasm — no matter how they started off. They have been aged anywhere from 30 to well over 70 years old.'

Tips

• Trying to teach yourself could result in injury.

• You'll need to take some lessons to get you off to the right start.

• Check out Nordic Walking organisations to link with other walkers, learn more about the sport and hear of upcoming events.

PROFILE

Nordic walking perfect ingredient for lifestyle recipe

Annabelle White is a cook, food writer, celebrity foodie and very active woman without her Nordic Walking poles; with them she says she is 'darn nearly invincible'. She fell in love with her new sport pretty much as soon as she discovered it four years ago, and on most days she is out the door for about an hour, striding up to 5 kilometres.

She was always a walker but she found adding poles to her walking brought numerous benefits. 'It's a brilliant workout, and certainly I went down a dress size. But it's more than a workout to me. It's my special time for both body and mind.' She likes to walk solo to de-stress from busy work days and to energise herself for the next one. She says the sticks bring less obvious benefits for the sole walker powering along on autopilot.

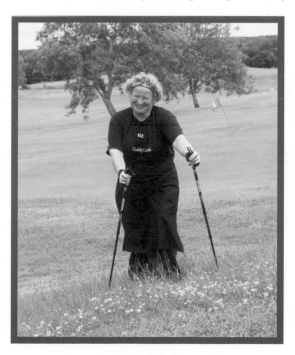

Annabelle White out with her walking poles in Ireland.

'They create a kind of private zone around you. You know no one is going to mess with you. And they leave you free to look around more because you're not so preoccupied with picking your way around hazards and obstacles. I feel more sure-footed with them. If you trip, the chances are the poles will help to save you.

'They do good things for my posture, too, and all round I feel more powerful.'

Annabelle is well aware that Nordic walkers are not a common sight and that some women may hesitate to take up this form of exercise for fear of ridicule.

'The only people who might think you look silly are those who haven't been around enough to know that this sport is huge in Europe with people of all ages. Not that I would care if people thought I looked daft when I am out walking. I think I am lucky to have discovered Nordic walking. I absolutely love it. No matter how I feel when I set off, I always return home feeling better.'

When she travels, those Nordic poles are in the luggage and she has been known to pop up with them, out and about in faraway places. Eager to spread the word on her new-found sport, the irrepressible Annabelle did a quick demo of Nordic walking on national television, where she is resident chef on a breakfast show.

PROFILE

Pushing into healthy old age with walking poles

'I feel on top of the world if I have been for a good walk.'

Jenny is the inspiration behind the enthusiastic group of Nordic-walking women in their 60s and 70s who have become affectionately known at events as the Nordic Nanas.

Taking up Nordic walking has brought a list of benefits for Jenny. Her posture has improved, back and neck problems are much lessened, it always boosts her mood, and it has brought a number of new, active friends into her life. It has also brought good things for the other women she has enlisted to join her in her new-found passion.

Jenny encountered Nordic walking five years ago at an expo on positive aging, when she was 67 years old and keen to find new ways to enhance her wellbeing.

'After a quick trial with the poles I was immediately hooked, and I knew it was right for me. The benefits were exactly what I needed and I loved the feeling walking with the poles gave me. And what's more, I thought I had a very good chance of being able to do it well enough to really get going.'

Jenny didn't have much of an exercise track-record to launch from, only a bit of line dancing and some tramping. She had had her share of back troubles and never been much of a sportsperson, although she knew that sport was good for health. Like so many women her age, she had done hours of service in sport as a 'sideline mum', taking care of mountains of laundry and cutting up oranges to hand around at half-time. But she figured it was never too late to get going, and now she had found the catalyst that would make her do it: those 'power along' poles! Embracing her new sport with great commitment from day one, Jenny quickly decided she wanted others to enjoy it — and to join her on regular walks.

She successfully sought funding from local government recreation coffers for a group of women to get walking poles and be taught how to use them. She also succeeded in getting local media to back her by spreading the word on the benefits of the sport and promoting it to older women in the region. Before long the Nordic Nanas were over a dozen strong and were regularly turning up to take part in walking events.

For Jenny, launching herself off on the walking poles was relatively easy after a bit of coaching and practice. But getting a regular group of walking women up and going took lots of determination and hard work. To get funding from the city council she sought the support of the residents' committee of the large retirement village she lives in to help her through the application process. With the first grant in 2007 she was able to buy 10 pairs of poles and pay a coach to deliver a six-week Nordic walking course from the retirement village.

Getting others to join was slow at first, but she had soon recruited around 15 novice walkers with the support of local newspaper stories and by pounding the pavements herself to deliver flyers to a thousand houses in the neighbourhood. A couple more grants in the following years helped fund more promotion and coaching, until the Acacia Grove Nordic Walkers became firmly established. Looking back, she says the job was far bigger than she had expected, bringing with it lots of paperwork, administration and many hours of her time. But today she says she is hooked, with a much invigorated life and a widened circle of friends.

The Nordic Nanas walk for an hour every Sunday and often during the week. If there is a half-marathon coming up, training cranks up to at least four days a week and sometimes the girls are out walking for three hours at a stretch.

In 2009 the Nordic Nanas did their first half-marathon together, with five of the 15-strong group in their 70s. It was some achievement, and not surprisingly these women turned a few heads at the time on the race day.

'I'd never imagined myself doing something like this. I'd had back surgery, back pain and a few problems with joints. I had no idea I could ever walk as far as I can now. And I can't tell you how good it makes me feel. When I have been for a good walk, I feel on top of the world. I would never stop now. It has been a lot of hard work to make our group such a success but if I can do it, others can do it too in their neighbourhoods. We are really proud of our group and the way we have really built up our walking.'

Chapter 13

WALKING YOUR FIRST HALF-MARATHON

Once you have become a regular walker and covered a fair few kilometres, you will be feeling the benefits of it and be quite easily able to step out for good long walks, of around 10 kilometres or so. You will have built up your fitness and found your weak spots. You could now be up for more of a challenge.

Maybe you started out pretty cautiously on the 10-week walking plan we used earlier in this book, from the Wonder Walkers website. If you did that, you'll have some idea of how you build your fitness and distance and all-round ability to walk further by making the commitment to a training plan and sticking to it. Maybe you've already entered a number of 5- and 10-kilometre fun walks.

Already you will have noticed that half-marathon events are scheduled regularly all year round. Plenty are happening somewhere near you, giving you a good range of choices for training and preparation, and for getting a walking buddy to work with you.

Stepping up to the challenge of walking a half-marathon can be great fun. It's exciting to set a goal that until recently you could not have imagined reaching. The distance is 21 kilometres, and reasonably fit walkers can do that distance in around four hours — give or take a bit. Nevertheless, walking 21 kilometres is not easy and that is why it is a challenge. It is a lot further than what you may have thought of as long walks to this point, but you will make it if you train well, and you will feel a real sense of achievement when you have done it.

Getting into training

Experts say doing the training is the thing. Ideally you will be starting your training around 12 weeks before the event and you will already have a basic level of fitness and be able to walk at a steady pace for at least 30 minutes four days a week. If this is the position you are starting from, you can embark on a realistic schedule that will take you across the finish line in reasonable time and in reasonable shape.

The training period to get into half-marathon condition really is not very long, and sticking to the schedule over the prescribed number of days and distances is the simple formula for success. Whatever the weather, you have to get out there and get used to it. After all, marathon day might be wet and windy.

Setting your schedule

It is easy enough to find a training schedule on the internet, and they have a similarity and a common goal. They provide you with a tried and tested plan (based on health and fitness science) that will build you up, progressively introducing longer walks in the weekly schedule. Some training plans do not go the whole 21 kilometres in the build-up. That is because it is assumed you will make it on the day quite easily, based on the training you have done and the excitement of the event. Others take the approach that covering the full distance in the training gives a great boost to being confident that you can make it on the day.

Our schedule was prepared for Wonder Walkers by one of the site's fitness experts, Wendy Sweet.

This training schedule is designed for first-timers and requires you to focus on increasing your distance for up to eight weeks before the event. The schedule aims to gradually increase your tolerance to the distance of a half-marathon. There is no focus on time or speed. You will need to have sturdy walking shoes (worn in, but not worn out) and loose clothing. Whatever your size, try to get some Lycra shorts or tights for walking the longer distances, so your skin doesn't get chafed. And don't forget a supportive bra.

The concept of training for a half-marathon is that you are gradually overloading your heart, lungs and legs over a set period of time in order to cope on the day. Each week you add extra distance (duration) to your longer walk. An increase of around 10 per cent can be generally tolerated by most beginner walkers each week. Days of training are also matched by some rest days to allow recovery time. The notion of training also means that as much as possible you need to replicate the conditions you will endure on the day. This includes knowing as much as you can about the type of terrain you will face, your water intake and timing, your food intake and timing and of course, your shoes and clothing.

I have written three paces for this programme: easy, moderate and fast. Experiment with the one you feel most comfortable with. Choose flat terrain at first if you are a little unfit, and, once you feel comfortable, move to more undulating terrain. Hills will really make you work harder, and these are great to add in at about the three- to four-week mark. Cutting back on your distance in the last week of this programme enables you to conserve vital energy in the days leading up to the half-marathon.

Mark out some fun 5-, 10- and 20-kilometre routes around your area before commencing your programme. This will enable you to plan ahead and to know exactly what you have to achieve in terms of the distance you have to cover. Take an extra rest day if you need to in the early weeks. Remember, too, that swimming or aqua-jogging is great non-impact recovery and flexibility training to add into your rest days. It would only take 20 minutes in the pool to aid your recovery from week to week.

Fast pace: Almost like a power walk, but not breaking into a jog. You should be breathing heavier than normal.

Moderate pace: You should be breathing heavier than normal, but still able to hold a conversation.

Easy pace: No stopping, but just enjoy the walk at a comfortable place. Easy pace is also used to recover after a harder session the day before.

NOTE: In the following tables, three choices are given for each day. Choose the programme that suits your personal fitness and goals.

Week 1

Goals: To build your distance and fitness gradually. To challenge the pace each time so that you have adequate recovery time between sessions. Beginner walkers may take one extra rest day if they require this week. Distances are given in kilometres.

WEEK ONE			
DAY 1	Walk 2 km *Easy*	Walk 2 km *Easy*	Walk 2 km *Easy*
DAY 2	Walk 2.5 km *Moderate*	Walk 3 km *Fast*	Walk 3.5 km *Moderate*
DAY 3	Rest	Rest	Rest
DAY 4	Walk 3 km *Moderate*	Walk 5 km *Moderate*	Walk 3 km *Fast*
DAY 5	Rest	Walk 3.5 km *Moderate*	Jog or fast walk 2 km
DAY 6	Walk 6 km *Easy*	Walk 3 km *Fast*	Walk 6 km *Moderate*
DAY 7	Rest	Rest	Rest

Week 2

Goals: To keep building strength and stamina for the distance you will need to cover later. By adding in some hills to your terrain this week, you will add strength to your legs and arms and you will also push your fitness up another notch.

WEEK TWO			
DAY 1	Walk 6 km *Moderate*	Walk 4 km *Fast*	Walk/Jog 5 km *Moderate/ Fast*
DAY 2	Walk 3 km *Moderate*	Walk 3.5 km *Moderate*	Walk 3.5 km *Moderate*
DAY 3	Rest	Rest	Rest
DAY 4	Walk 3 km *Easy**	Walk 3 km *Fast*	Fast walk/Jog 3 km
DAY 5	Walk 2 km *Fast*	Walk 4 km *Easy hilly*	Jog 3 km *Easy hilly*
DAY 6	Walk 10 km *Easy hilly*	Walk 6 km *Moderate*	Walk 10 km *Easy*
DAY 7	Rest	Rest	Rest

* Add some mixed terrain here. Flat to start, then some gentle hills.

Week 3

Goals: To keep building strength and stamina for the distance as well as some faster-paced walking/jogging to get you ready for the pace you need to do on the day of the event.

WEEK THREE			
DAY 1	Walk 6 km Moderate/ Fast	Walk 5 km Moderate	Fast walk/Jog 3 km
DAY 2	Walk 5 km Moderate	Walk 5 km Easy hilly	Walk/Easy jog 10 km
DAY 3	Rest	Rest	Rest
DAY 4	Walk 4 km Easy	Walk 4 km Fast	Race pace walk 5 km
DAY 5	Walk 5 km Fast	Walk 2 km Easy/Fast hilly	Walk 8 km Easy
DAY 6	Rest	Walk 8 km Moderate	Walk 15 km Moderate
DAY 7	Walk 15 km Easy	Rest	Rest

Week 4

Goals: To start focusing on the event and get you faster for event day, as well as building your strength with continued hill work.

WEEK FOUR			
DAY 1	Walk 6 km Moderate/ Fast	Walk 8 km Easy	Fast walk/Jog 3 km
DAY 2	Rest	Walk 5 km Easy hilly	Walk 8 km Moderate
DAY 3	Walk 10 km Moderate	Rest	Rest
DAY 4	Walk 6 km Easy	*Walk 2 km Fast	*Walk 5 km Fast
DAY 5	Rest	Walk 5 km Easy/ Moderate	*Walk/jog 8 km Moderate
DAY 6	Walk 15 km Easy/ Moderate	Rest	Rest
DAY 7	Rest	Walk 10 km Moderate/ Easy	Walk 17 km Easy

*Complete this session over the course if you can.

Week 5

Goals: To complete the course at race pace, and keep building your speed and distance covered, based on your fitness level.

WEEK FIVE			
DAY 1	Walk 5 km *Easy*	Rest	Slow jog 5 km *Easy*
DAY 2	Walk 3 km *Fast*	Walk 16 km *Easy hilly*	Walk 10 km *Moderate
DAY 3	Rest	Rest	Rest
DAY 4	Walk 15 km	Walk 3 km *Fast*	Rest
DAY 5	Walk 2 km *Fast*	Walk 8 km *Moderate* on course	Walk 15 km *Easy/ Moderate*
DAY 6	Walk 5 km *Moderate*	Rest	Walk 5 km *Easy*
DAY 7	Rest	Walk 10 km *Easy*	Rest

*Complete this section at the pace you want to do on the day of the event. Use the course if you can, so that psychologically you know that you can get through the event on the day.

Week 6

Goals: To keep building your distance covered over the next week so that you are hitting the 21 kilometres. This is a crucial psychological boost so that you know you can complete the event two weeks out.

WEEK SIX			
DAY 1	Walk 8 km *Easy*	Rest	Slow jog 5 km *Easy*
DAY 2	Walk 3 km *Fast*	Walk 16 km *Easy hilly*	Walk 12 km *Moderate**
DAY 3	Rest, swim, stretch, rest		
DAY 4	Walk 15 km*	Walk 3 km *Fast*	Rest, swim, stretch
DAY 5	Rest	Walk 20 km (*Moderate** on course) **or** Walk 20 km (*Easy/Moderate*)	
DAY 6	Walk 20 km *Easy/ Moderate*	Rest	Walk 5 km *Easy hilly*
DAY 7	Rest	Walk 10 km *Easy*	Rest

*This is a big jump in distance this week so ensure that you have the time to do the longer distance at your own pace. You will need to carry extra water/glucose drink and have some nutrition bars/fruit on you when you are doing the longer distance.

Week 7

Goals: This week is the same as the previous week, but add one more kilometre on to your long walk so that you know you have done the distance a good week out from the event. This is also a time for you to keep practising the timing of your food and fluid intake as you complete the long walks.

WEEK SEVEN		
DAY 1	Walk 8 km *Easy*	Rest	Slow jog 5 km *Easy*
DAY 2	Walk 3 km *Fast*	Walk 16 km *Easy hilly*	Walk 12 km *Moderate**
DAY 3	Rest, swim, stretch, rest, swim, stretch, rest		
DAY 4	Walk 15 km*	Walk 3 km *Fast*	Rest, swim, stretch
DAY 5	Rest	Walk 21 km (*Moderate** on course) **or** Walk 20 km (*Easy/Moderate*)	
DAY 6	Walk 21 km *Easy/ Moderate*	Rest	Walk 5 km *Easy hilly*
DAY 7	Rest	Walk 10 km *Easy*	Rest

*For this extra distance make sure you carry extra water/glucose drink and some nutrition bars/fruit with you.

Week 8

Goals: To keep your pace up but cut back the distances, so that you are fresh for the day of the event. This week is called a 'taper week'.

WEEK EIGHT			
DAY 1	Rest	Walk 3 km *Moderate*	Rest
DAY 2	Walk 15 km *Easy*	Walk 21 km (*Moderate** on course) **or** Walk 20 km (*Easy/Moderate*)	
DAY 3	Rest	Rest	Rest
DAY 4	Walk 8 km *Easy*	Walk 8 km *Easy*	Walk/Jog 8 km *Moderate*
DAY 5	Walk 5 km *Moderate*	Walk 5 km *Moderate*	Walk/Jog 2 km *Moderate*
DAY 6	Walk 2 km *Easy*	Walk 1 km *Fast*	Walk/Jog 1.5 km *Fast*
DAY 7	**THE BIG EVENT DAY**		

Getting organised the day before

Pack everything you need. Drink extra water over the afternoon. Eat healthy foods and keep snacking right up to bedtime on low-fat snacks so you are well loaded up with energy. Go to bed in time to get a good night's sleep.

On marathon day

- Eat a normal breakfast, but not too much high fibre or you'll be looking for toilets on the route.
- Drink a bit of extra water and double check that you have packed all you need according to the personal food and fluid requirements you will have worked out during training — including your water bottle.
- If the weather is bad, you will have to layer and work out how to gather up the things later that you peel off along the way, as you will surely need to.

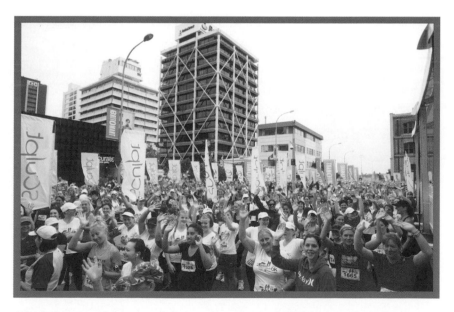

A large group of women about to start the Sculpt Women's 6k event in Auckland. *Photo Marathon-Photos.*

PROFILE

Late starter getting the best from distance walking

Noema Williams is the principal of a primary school in a rural area, where there are about 90 children enrolled.

At an age when a school principal might be dreaming of retirement and a quieter life, Noema's life runs at full steam, and outside the school gates she has set herself a pretty daunting schedule. Relatively late in life she challenged herself to get into better shape, through both exercise and walking — and a good dollop of commitment. Knowing a bit about leading the way and about motivating others, Noema went looking for her own special mentor and she put herself in the hands of a personal trainer, Sue Price — a dedicated fitness guru who in 2009 was named New Zealand's top personal trainer. Sue was exactly the right leader for Noema, who, credits Sue for giving her the guidance to becoming fitter and healthier and for keeping her on track.

Noema says she thinks a lot when she walks, and the subject of leadership both in life and the workplace is something she's given a lot of thought to: 'I think leadership is about many people and comes from many places. It is about learning, and it's about the sharing of knowledge. When I share my knowledge with others, they can then take up the challenge — like a flock of birds in migration — each can take a lead.'

In her own words, Noema Williams tells about getting fit and getting out there in later life:

> I am a Maori woman, 65 years young. I am a diabetic (Type 2) and I have been so for the past eight years. I am fit and my weight is in proportion to my height. I ensure that I have a nutritionally balanced diet; after all, I need to for the sake of my long-term health. I am in full-time, highly paid employment. I have no desire to retire anytime soon!

I am a child off a farm in the backblocks. Although our family was fortunate to own a motor vehicle, my brothers and I walked (mostly ran) everywhere out of sheer necessity really — to get cows in for milking, sheep in for shearing, feeding pigs and to get the school bus. So I generally maintained a moderately active lifestyle. That is, until I began walking/ running.

I was initially motivated about two years ago by the thought that if I maintained a regime of good nutrition and exercise, then, despite my diabetes, I would live to see my mokopuna (grandchildren). The other motivating factor was reading about a Hawaiian marathon where one competitor came in 12 hours after the start, and I thought 'Jeepers, I could do that too. I won't break any records, but I could still do it.' As an appetiser and just for fun, I entered a local marathon in 2008 along with eight members of my family. I was surprised that I completed it in three hours and five minutes. Not one of us had done anything like it before. And we could still walk afterwards.

So my mad thought turned into a desire to do the Auckland marathon in 2009 to celebrate the completion of the first draft of my PhD. I knew that I had to elevate my level of fitness. I was walking for about half an hour, sometimes for an hour. I thought I would walk the marathon.

I contacted a local personal trainer. On the first appointment she took blood pressure, weight, height and worked first on goals and an exercise plan for each day that I would be happy to carry through to achieve overall body fitness. The plan included (and still includes) strength and conditioning (cardio, shoulders, arms, legs, core) and for all the muscle groups and road running (and walking) to achieve mileage. She said to bring a bottle of water and a towel because I would sweat. God, I could barely walk after the first session! I was not even sure whether I should be elated. I had begun my journey. It was 11 months out from the marathon start.

Since December 2008 my personal trainer and I have met every six weeks or thereabouts. I would not be without one. The cost is minimal compared to the benefits I have accrued and will continue to gain for life. My personal trainer provides me with tools for fitness. But it is my task to do the work. No one else can do it for you.

I also visit my chiropractor every six weeks. Age has a way of creeping up on one. Some things occur as a natural part of aging, but I'd prefer to know about my old joints and bones sooner rather than later. I age with the knowledge and acceptance that I have the power to do something about most things. And it is okay to age gracefully.

For three months before (and also three months after) the marathon I pay monthly visits to the nutritionist. I work towards literally dumping the visceral fat around my tummy area through close attention to my nutritional needs. It's awesome. It has been difficult to build up muscle but I have, and it is imperative that I do so because I lost 3 kilograms of muscle on the 2009 marathon.

I am self-motivated and highly disciplined. I walk or run over some distance now (it is not unusual for me to walk for 21 kilometres on my Saturday walk), as well as maintain my exercise regime during the week. I look forward to walking long distances (must be the endorphins). I take sufficient water and fill my pockets with as many energy gel packs as I can. I walk through beautiful countryside where there is, for the most part, no one else but me.

As I go, I do a great deal of thinking — about life in general, my personal and work goals, books, theories and practices, about what motivates me and really how fortunate I am to enjoy the luxury of good health and a good brain. I live very much by the motto 'use it or lose it', and learn from and enjoy every waking moment. Walking helps me to do just that.

I love to walk and walking loves me.

Chapter 14

WALKING ABROAD: INTERNATIONAL MARATHONS AND WALKING HOLIDAYS

Serious walking these days takes lots of women a long way from home in the name of challenge, adventure and fun. More and more are flying off to some of the world's great walks for incredible holidays or taking part in international marathons. Many who have started off walking with friends close to home have found themselves getting much more ambitious, planning, saving and training for much bigger adventures, far from home. Depending on available time and budget, there is a tremendous range of well-charted walking routes and a growing list of marathons on offer all over the world for groups and those adventurous women who are happy to go it alone.

Walking international marathons

Not everyone is a runner, and many international marathons and half-marathons now welcome walkers and keep the course open long enough for the walkers to cross the finishing line and collect their medals well after the runners have finished. Most months of the year somewhere in the world there is a marathon or half-marathon you could turn into a memorable personal challenge and holiday combined. There are walker-friendly events to be found all year round in the United States, Europe and Australia, most have informative websites and make finding a marathon experience to suit your needs relatively easy. Some travel agents specialise in putting together marathon packages.

The big city events are very popular, though, so you would need to look into registering at the one of your choice many months in advance, if not a year. Of course that gives you plenty of time to train before taking off with other women, young and not so young, who are giving marathons a go all over the world.

Top walker-friendly marathons

• Dublin (October)
• Chicago (October)
• New York City (November)
• Honolulu (December)
• Los Angeles City (March)
• London (April)
• Vancouver (May)

These are just the big city marathons, and each has its own history and prestige. However, if you want to combine a marathon walk with an overseas trip, you probably won't have to search far to find one to fit into your schedule in the United States or in Europe.

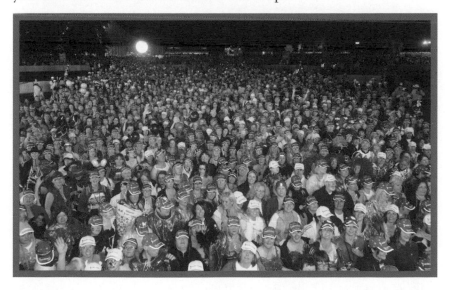

A sea of starters out at midnight for London's MoonWalk. *Photo Walk the Walk.*

The MoonWalk fund-raisers for breast cancer are attracting more and more entrants since they first started in London 15 years ago and have raised over £65 million. They begin at midnight and are a fabulous spectacle as well as a moving experience for entrants. The events are well supported by colourful themes, and many of the entrants wear elaborately decorated bras.

• MoonWalk London (May)
• MoonWalk Edinburgh (June)
• MoonWalk Iceland (June)

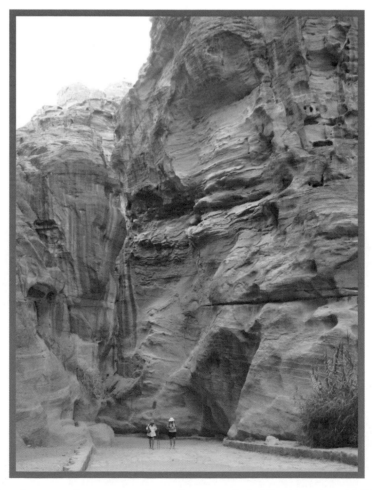

Walking the gorge in Petra, Jordan. *Photo Frank Goldingham, NZ Walking magazine*

Overseas walking holidays

Walking holidays around the world have become hugely popular, and there are many websites and travel specialists offering a wealth of information, making it easy to turn dreams into well-thought-out plans. While of course it is perfectly possible to simply set off and walk almost anywhere in the world that takes your fancy, it is also now possible to browse the net at home or let the experts guide you to the sort of experience you are looking for specifically. Seasons, distance, available time, budget, required level of fitness, accommodation choices, good advice, well-researched information, and the stories of those who have walked that way before you are only a key stroke or telephone call away.

The selection of well-charted walking packages is mind-boggling, and the regions on offer include Europe, India, Morocco, South America, North America, China, India, Egypt and Australia. And those are just the popular well-trodden routes, which more and more people are discovering on foot. Many are trips that can be done by allowing just two to three weeks away from home. For a taste of walking in Australia, of course, a week or so away would be viable for a great walking holiday.

Choosing the right walk

While travel experts and websites on world walks can be found in many places, there are a number of organisations where specialists in this sort of trip have helped many happy adventurers put together very memorable trips — without encountering half the snags they might have stumbled over by going it all alone.

One of the older hands in researching and compiling walking holidays is Jill Grant at Walker's World in Auckland. She was lured into it by a postcard from an intrepid aunt on a walking holiday in Switzerland, with tales of gourmet food, wonderful scenery, comfortable beds and people to help with luggage. That was over 20 years ago, but it inspired Jill to explore the market for people who might also like that sort of overseas walking holiday. A keen walker, Jill was much more familiar with the Kiwi way of hard-slog tramping, crowded tramping huts, hard bunks, basic food and the all-round discomfort that can become a lot less attractive with age — or when there are more attractive ways to do things.

Turning her passion into a business has included doing many walks in a range of countries, and compiling detailed notes giving clients useful information and tips on the ground. Most clients want to walk independently, but value the backup they receive from the 'footloose' packages. Commonly, this style of trip includes pre-booked accommodation on a bed-and-breakfast basis, local contacts and luggage transfers, plus detailed walking notes and route maps.

According to Jill, many newcomers to this style of travel get so much out of the experience they are soon planning another trip. For some of the women she packs off in little groups, the trip is a celebration of one of those milestone birthdays whether they are turning 40, 50, 60 or even 70. Along with physical challenge, they are looking for adventure, history, the experience of other cultures, a real change of scenery and, of course, very memorable fun.

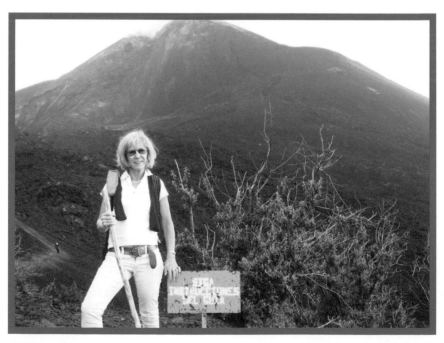

Jill Grant in Guatemala.

Popular overseas walking choices

• Italy's Cinque Terre
• The Amalfi Coast
• Mt Blanc
• The Inca Trail
• The Camino de Santiago/Way of St James
• The Danube Pathway
• Tuscany Trails
• Provence
• Croatia
• The Great Ocean Walk (Victoria, Australia)
• The Coast to Coast (Britain)
• The Amber Trail (Budapest)

People choose these international walking holidays for all sorts of reasons, and they can be seeking different types of experiences — and challenges. Some want culture and history, some love the landscapes and scenery, some dream of great food and wine, while others could be looking for the challenge of a lifetime.

'Deciding what you are looking for is important when there are now so many walks to choose from. With a bit of research you get the best. But a bit of realism is important, too — we certainly don't want to be sending people off on trips they are not fit enough for or that are not within their capabilities.'

'People need to be realistic about the choosing the right seasons, too, or they can find extremes of weather and temperatures turn the dream into a nightmare trip they would rather forget. They also need to understand how much time they need to allow for their walks, allowing for the effects of a long flight to the starting point. And of course they also need to be realistic about getting physically prepared.'

Jill has a wealth of advice, but these are a few tips for making the most of a walking holiday overseas:

- Take a spirit of adventure — there are no guarantees.
- Do not skimp on walking shoes: wear ankle boots, not trainers. Going over on an ankle can ruin that trip.
- Fitness is critical — do the preparation.
- Do not underestimate the challenge.
- Invest in the right clothes for the conditions.
- Read the walking notes and information.

A taste of popular walks in various countries

The Camino de Santiago: The Way of St James

This one is the biggie in overseas walking holidays, but it can also be done in selected small bits if time and other demands are pressing. The full route to the shrine of St James is 800 kilometres, and it takes from at least a month to six weeks to complete the journey.

The pilgrim's way in Spain has a very old history as the much-travelled route across northern Spain for the literally millions of pilgrims who travelled it many centuries ago. It is still a pilgrim route today, although lots of the ancient pathways have been wiped out by highways and development. The appeal of following this trunk road of the 12th and 13th centuries is still very much alive. In recent times it has had a big revival and attracts walkers bent on journeys both long and short.

The best times to go are in the northern hemisphere spring and autumn months for the ideal walking weather. A good level of fitness is required, as this route is mostly over hilly terrain. The days on foot are long. On many days walkers cover around 24 kilometres, but sometimes that can be up to 33 kilometres.

The trip starts either at the Roncesvalles Pass on the Spanish side of the Pyrénées or at Saint-Jean-Pied-de Port on the French side. The main trail is through Puente la Reina, La Rioja, Burgos, León and then crosses Galicia to finish in medieval city of Santiago de Compostela in northwest Spain.

Much of what moved the thousands of pilgrims also moves the modern-day walkers as a profound and quite spiritual experience — as well as a standout holiday and physical tone-up.

If you can't do it in one go, it is quite possible to do a week or eight days' walking from various points along the way. Some people do this, until they have joined up their stages to complete the entire journey.

The walk passes through lush valleys, over bridges, through countless charming villages, forests, streams and past many, many, fine historical buildings. Overnight lodgings for the stream of walkers through these parts include monasteries and convents that have been revamped for a new lease of life, as well as historic inns and bed-and-breakfast establishments.

For a short walk on the pilgrim's way, some suggest the earlier sections, which will be quieter than joining the throng on the last leg to the home of the shrine. Many choose to do the last 100 kilometres of the walkway to experience the thrill of entering the city of their destination on foot. There they have the unforgettable experience of joining the crowds for mass at Santiago de Compestela's beautiful cathedral where the remains of St James the Great are believed to lie.

The Great Ocean Walk, Victoria, Australia

In recent years this has become a very popular long-distance walk on the southwest coast of Victoria, and, although it is possible to walk it independently, there are plenty of packages available for various options and various budgets and levels of accommodation.

The Great Ocean Walk is about 104 kilometres long and is located between the Great Ocean Road and the sea. The start point is 200 kilometres west from Melbourne, at Apollo Bay, and the route runs west to finish in the vicinity of the spectacular rock stacks known as the 12 Apostles. But you don't have to walk all the way (or back) at once. The route is designed for walkers to be able to step on and off easily at many points. At the most basic end of comfort there are about seven campsites to choose from, but there are also purpose-built lodges, cabins and other accommodation en route for walkers. There are also towns and settlements to stop off at, along the way.

Depending on fitness and weather, the entire walk takes at least five days and often up to 10 days. There is a range of choice for walkers to plan how far and how fast they go, the standard of overnight stops and how much emphasis they want to put on food, wine and provisioning. You can do it with a touch of luxury and rest for a day or two, or you can make this walkway as much of a challenge as you like!

As well as magnificent coastal scenery, the walk offers so much of what is uniquely Australian — surf beaches, wallabies, koalas, snakes, birds and insects, national parklands and rainforest. The 12 Apostles rising up out of the ocean are a magnificent sight at the end of the journey.

Cinque Terre, Italy

This is a very long-established walk along a rugged section of coastline that's been well trodden by many visitors to Italy. It is in Liguria in the northwest of the country. Cinque Terre is Italian for 'five lands', which refers to the five small coastal villages that are connected by the walking trails.

All but one of the towns slope down to sea level. The pathways between the towns pass through great natural scenery, good swimming beaches and exhilarating views. The little villages are Riomaggiore (the southernmost town), Manarola, Corniglia, Vernazza and Monterosso al Mare. The latter is the northernmost town and is much more of a resort town with the least charm of all. The others have all the appeal of Italian villages, from little winding streets and beautiful old houses to pretty fishing fleets, an abundance of culture and history, many cafés and marketplaces and, of course, all that tasty Italian fare that is part of any holiday in this country.

A good level of fitness is required because, although some of the going is relatively easy, there are plenty of hill climbs (and descents) and many, many steps. There is a tough, steep section from Vernazza to Monterosso, where walkers must clamber for quite a distance over very uneven rocks.

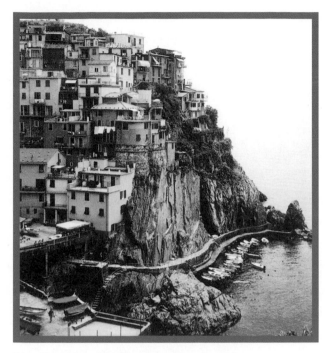

The picturesque pathway at Riomaggiore.

The walks between villages take the best part of a day. In high summer temperatures it is necessary to start out early in order to avoid a trying hour or so in the heat of the day. Although there are many inns, hotels and bed-and-breakfast places in every town, a booking is essential (in the high season at least) or a long, hot day could well end with a long, hot trudge around the village in search of a place to spend the night.

This is a walk you can structure to do at your own pace (if you set off early enough each day). You can rest as long as you like at any village along the way, and you can skip the toughest sections if you choose.

The Amalfi Coast, Italy

This is coastal walk in southern Italy that has become very popular. The route follows ancient walking paths between Ravello and Positano, a distance that can be covered in about a week with a rest day along the way. It is high above the sea and calls for a good level of fitness. Most days you would be walking between village and countryside, with plenty of steps and hill work on the way. There are wonderful views and plenty of Italian hospitality to be enjoyed at the end of the day. There is a range of accommodation to suit most budgets in the handful of villages you pass through.

The Inca Trail, Peru

The Inca Trail is the most famous hiking or walking route in South America and it's an experience many an adventurous soul has high up on their 'to do one day' list. This trail takes you to one of the new Seven Wonders of the World, the site of the ruins of Machu Picchu, lost city of the Incas. More of a hike than a walk, you need to be fit and wear strong shoes or boots.

The trail to Machu Picchu is about 45 kilometres long and the journey takes four days, including a day spent exploring the ruins. From there, walkers can travel back to the town of Cusco by train.

Although the views of mountains and forest are stunning, the walking route is steep and demanding in parts, rising up from valleys and over particularly over high passes. On the way to Machu Picchu there is also plenty to see of archaeological interest.

As both Peru, and Machu Picchu in particular, are a bit off the beaten track, this is a walk that will need planning beyond merely getting fit and equipped to do it. It also needs to be booked, because the number of walkers allowed here is controlled.

It is important to take into account that this is a walk in high altitudes, the likes of which you may never have encountered before. Altitude sickness is a risk for walkers and, as anyone who has been hit by it knows, it could ruin your trip. Unfortunately, there is no way of knowing in advance if you will be susceptible to it, so it is best to build in preparations to ward it off. To combat the possibility of being hit by altitude sickness, travellers are advised to arrive in the region at least a few days before they set off walking so that they have some time to gradually acclimatise to the higher altitude. Ignore this precaution at your peril!

The Inca Trail is closed in February, but otherwise open. The best time to walk it is in the dry season, between April and October. The wet season runs from November to March.

Walking in Britain: The Coast to Coast path

Walking or rambling (as the English often call it) is a very popular holiday choice in the beautiful British countryside. But many an outdoors-loving traveller is very grateful to the foresight and vision of Alfred Wainwright, the intrepid walker who thought of mapping the route that in 1972 became Britain's lovely Coast to Coast walk. It is a long-distance footpath of 308 kilometres running from west coast to east, across the Lake District, the Yorkshire Dales and the North York Moors. It has been well planned to cross through some of the country's finest scenery, ensuring its appeal both with the English and walkers from many other countries.

The Coast to Coast starts beside the Irish Sea, at the town of St Bees and there are many towns and hamlets to pass through or explore as you walk. The establishment of this walking path has not only been an attractive drawcard for walkers, but also a boon for all those businesses, from travel organisations to the inns and eateries, both large and small, who provide the all-important supporting cast. Because it is such a long walk, not all who take to the paths can spend weeks on their rambling holiday, and some just drop in and out at various points, arranging accommodation and routes to suit their available time, stamina and budget.

The townships along the route are comfortably spaced for a day-walk of about 15 kilometres, or for shorter stints on less energetic days. Some of these towns are more remote and quite sparsely populated. The route at times takes in some lonely, albeit beautiful, territory and, although it is possible to go alone, walkers usually go in pairs or groups.

A good standard of fitness is required to sustain the long days, and some of the terrain is more challenging in places. However, distances and challenges can be taken into account when planning the trip and well before you embark on it.

Weather in the region is unpredictable, even in the summery months from May to September. Walkers have to be prepared to cope with anything from heavy rain, high winds and cold days to glorious hot weather and the risk of sunburn. The good news is that in mid-summer days are long in this part of the world — it is light before 5am and night doesn't fall until nearly 10pm. That is a lot of possible walking hours per day if you are taking your time on the long hauls.

There is accommodation available from budget to high end and what you budget to spend during the walking days is up to you.

For the terrain and distance, boots are advised, plus a back-up pair of walking shoes.

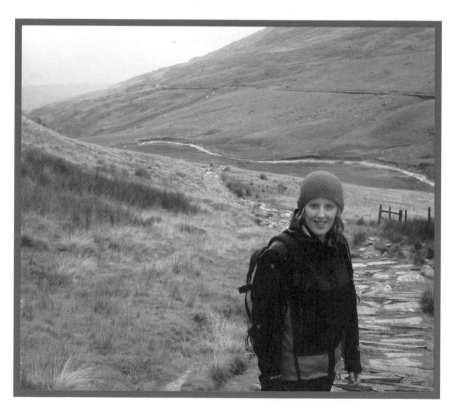

A young walker dressed for a wet walk on Mt Snowdon in Wales.

Other highly rated walks in Britain

• South West Coast Path

• Pennine Way

• Southern Upland Way

• Hadrian's Wall Path

• The Ridgeway

• Land's End to John O'Groats

• South Downs Way

• South West Coast National Trail

• Pembrokeshire Coast Trail

Walking in New Zealand

There is a tremendous range of spectacular walking on offer in New Zealand through magnificent scenery. Walkers and hikers of all levels of fitness can choose to explore mountains, forests, and coastline on an array of very well-maintained tracks, according to preference, from gentle day walks to multi-day treks over more challenging and remote terrain.

The big walks are to be found well away from the cities and larger towns, but all regions have well-marked walking routes where it is easy enough to put together a memorable few hours or a day of walking through forest or over coastline.

Adventure tourism in the outdoors is popular with both locals and the worldwide walking fraternity alike. The country's widely known big walks or great walks number about a dozen, and most are located in the South Island. The Milford Track is probably the best known, but all on this list are maintained to a high standard by the government, and they are a magnet in the summer season for serious walkers from all corners of the world. And while they may be labelled 'walks', they are really hikes that are quite challenging just by virtue of the fact that they traverse remote mountains and forests in a very capricious climate. In a heartbeat, high summer can give way to high winds, rain and dramatic drops in temperature.

In short, the great multi-day walks call for at least moderate fitness, preparation and good gear. The features and demands of them all are well documented on dedicated websites.

All of the great walks require booking ahead, particularly for freedom walkers who will be sleeping and self-catering in the basic but comfortable huts en route. To freedom walk the very popular Milford Track, for example, it is necessary to book almost a year in advance. The southernmost of the tracks are only open from November to April.

If freedom walking with heavy packs and 'ready for anything' clothing and equipment seems too daunting, most have guided options where gear is carried for you and dinner awaits in comfortable quarters at the end of each big day.

Top multi-day walks/hikes — South Island

The Milford Track: Claimed by many to be the finest walk in the world, this trek crosses the mountains and lush rainforests of Fiordland National Park. Beginning at Lake Te Anau and finishing in Milford Sound, this is a four- to five-day hike of 53.5 kilometres.

The Routeburn Track: A two- to four-day walk of 32 kilometres. It crosses through both Mount Aspiring and Fiordland National Parks, and can be varied by including the Greenstone Track.

The Kepler Track: Also in Fiordland National Park, this is 60 kilometres and takes three to four days.

The Heaphy Track: The longest of these tracks at 78.4 kilometres. It is further north, in the Kahurangi National Park in the northwest of the South Island. You can walk the Heaphy Track all year round — weather permitting, of course.

Abel Tasman Coast Track: Located at the top of the South Island. This is one of the easier multi-day walks in the top selection. It is 51 kilometres and can be covered over three to five days. It includes beautiful coastline and great beaches and is open all year round.

The Queen Charlotte Track: This beautiful track offers softer options for those who like to have the choice of taking some of their walking holiday a little easier and with a little comfort, fine wine and good food to enhance to experience. You can go guided or walk independently, but if you tire of the challenge, it is possible to board a water taxi at some points and give your legs a rest. It is located in the Marlborough Sounds and can usually be walked all year round. It stretches for 71 kilometres and takes about four days.

Top multi-day walks/hikes — Central North Island

Lake Waikaremoana: This is a 46-kilometre track through pristine forest high in the rugged terrain of Te Urewera National Park. It can be walked with guides or independently from hut to hut, and takes from three to four days.

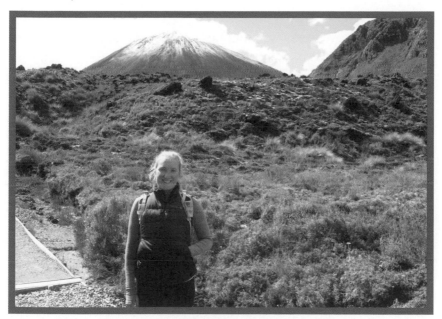

An Australian walker tackles the Tongariro Crossing one-day hike in New Zealand.

Tongariro: This is the volcanic central plateau of the North Island, with walking tracks through tussock grassland, across mountain slopes, past geysers, lava formations, and lakes which make this area quite unlike any other hiking region in New Zealand. It is possible to walk for at least a couple of days here, but the one-day walk known as the Tongariro Crossing is a popular track. It is no 'walk in the park', though, and you need to be fit for this challenging walk in exposed terrain where you are very much at the mercy of the weather. The track is just over 19 kilometres and takes from seven to nine hours' steady walking.

Austria: The Danube Pathway

This pathway has only recently been developed for all-year-round walking. It follows the valley of the Danube River offering about 450 kilometres of great walking along hillsides, through forests, meadows, very pretty villages with the traditional timbered houses, and many a castle and fortress. It runs from Passau to not far from Vienna. Most walkers, whether in organised groups or going independently, will do big days of 20 kilometres or more of relatively easy walking. Views of the Danube are a constant pleasure on this route through nature and history.

The two main stages on this pathway are from Passau to Linz and from Linz to Grein. The latter stage, ending in the historic town of Grein, is one of the prettiest stretches to walk. This can be covered in eight days by independent walkers.

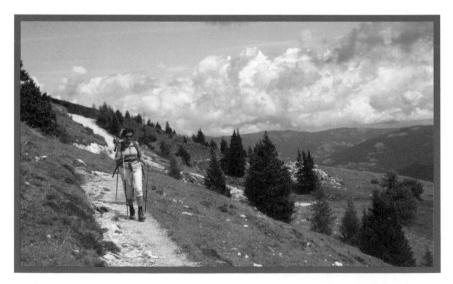

Walking in the Austrian Alps. *Photo Frank Goldingham, NZ Walking magazine*

France: Walking in Provence

Walking in France is very popular, and the country has tremendous networks of hiking trails and walking routes ranging from very challenging to easy-going. There are thousands of kilometres of pathways that link villages and offer wonderful rambling for days, weeks or even months.

For good reason, the Provence region in the south east of France is a magnet for an endless stream of walkers of all ages and fitness levels, because it offers a taste of most of the finer things in life — wonderful sights, good weather, great food and wine, endless charm, history and much more.

Some who explore this region on foot say it is easier logistically to base themselves in a village and make daily forays on different circular routes to various destinations and experiences, returning to the same place each night. Others choose to walk from village to village according to their own plans and well armed with good maps. Winter, spring and autumn are the best times for walking. However May is an especially nice time for walking in Provence, before the high hordes of holiday-makers crowd into the villages and the summer heat kicks in, necessitating early morning starts for adventures on foot.

The Luberon area, stretching along a rugged ridge of hills, foothills and countryside is a great destination for walkers, with an extensive network of accessible paths linking villages that are often just a few kilometres apart. If you avoid the mountains, you don't have to be super-fit or a serious hiker to enjoy exploring this region on foot.

The paths take you through farmland, vineyards, woods, orchards, past ancient buildings and landmarks, and sometimes climb to tiny villages perched on hilltops. How high or how far depends of the walking routes chosen from maps and guides that are readily available. For the most part, walking routes are well maintained. There is plenty of signage en route, but seasoned walkers in these parts advise you to carry maps rather than relying on the markers you find as you go.

Because it is so beautiful, this is a busy part of the world (unless you are off the beaten track), so advance planning is advised.

California: great walking places

There are many opportunities for walking on California's rugged Pacific coast, located within striking distance of Los Angeles and San Francisco.

Point Reyes

This is a national seashore preservation area under the wing of the US National Park Service. It is a prominent cape, just 50 kilometres west and north of San Francisco. You can walk for miles here on a choice of many trails, or just choose a half-day of walking on trails from easy to moderately challenging.

In total there are nearly 240 kilometres of walking and hiking trails at Point Reyes. The National Park Service website for this spectacular coastal wilderness lists and describes many of the trails and their entry points. They are grouped in walks of under an hour, one- to three-hour hikes, and three- to six-hour hikes which run for distances of from 15 to 20 kilometres. Although it is year-round walking, sections of some tracks can be closed in rough weather, but the Park Service's visitor centre makes it easy to get information about all routes.

Point Lobos State Reserve

Although the trails are not long here, the walks on this stunning coastal reserve are high on the national list of favourites in the United States. Point Lobos State Reserve is on the magnificent coastal highway route that runs between Los Angeles and San Francisco. It is in the Monterey region, south of the fabulous Monterey Bay aquarium, and the park entrance is about 5 kilometres south again of the charming township of Carmel.

There are many short tracks around the reserve, but a favourite is the perimeter track, which is a walk of around 10 kilometres. This passes beaches, coves, rocks and cliffs, and calls for good shoes and a degree of surefootedness. There are wildflowers and sea birds, seals and stunning wild ocean views. From March to May, walkers frequently see migrating whales. It can be pretty hot in high summer in this part of California, but that is often tempered by the fogs that roll in regularly from July to September.

The reserve is very popular and, because visitor numbers are restricted, it is best to avoid the busiest times.

Canada

The Bruce Trail and Niagara Falls

The Bruce Trail is 840 kilometres long and is one of the oldest in Canada. It follows the Niagara Escarpment, starting not far from the famous falls at the border of New York and Canada, and travels all the way up past Lake Ontario to the tip of the Bruce Peninsula. A hugely popular route with walkers and hikers, it attracts about 400,000 people a year to tread many different sections from various access points, but many start at the southern end, incorporating a separate visit to Niagara Falls nearby. For actually visiting the falls, there are a couple of options: a damp foray behind the falls, or suspended above the falls on a 325-kilometre boardwalk.

Naturally over such a long distance, the Bruce Trail passes through distinctly different regions. The southernmost section — starting nearest the falls — is a green corridor through southern Ontario. There are waterfalls aplenty and great views of Lake Ontario. The mid-section of the trail disappears into hillsides until it comes back out to follow along Georgian Bay, sometimes high up on the escarpment ledges.

PROFILE

Walking overseas: making it happen at 60

Sally Markham didn't get to take her first walking holiday in Europe until she had passed her 60th, but now — three walks and seven years later — she says she is 'hooked' on this way of exploring little sections of faraway places. An arts educator, with a very strong interest in history, she wanted her explorations to be about learning as well as fitness, walking and all the other benefits that special holidays bring.

For the trips she has taken every second year, she has chosen to follow the footsteps of pilgrims, and explore castles and remote villages in France and Spain.

After some research she chose the 'footloose'-style eight- to 10-day walk that appeals to so many of the people who want to go on walking holidays but have to fit it into busy lives and average budgets. While travel, accommodation and many other things are organised for you, on a day-to-day basis you are on your own or with your travelling companion only — these footloose walks are not guided. And while travelling 'footloose' can throw up a few challenges along the way, Sally says for her it is the perfect choice. 'You can do it your way, go at your own pace, and put the emphasis each day how you want it.'

For Sally, these walking holidays are affordable every second year with a bit of planning and saving. Although she is happy enough to be largely self-reliant on her walking trips, she wanted to minimise mishaps by taking the advice of those who had gone before her and to be as well informed and organised as they would advise. While not upmarket, accommodation and meals were comfortable and good quality — not to mention very memorable in some of the historic settings in which this walker has found herself.

Her first trip in 2005, with her son, was eight days of walking to the remains of the Cathar Castles in the Languedoc region of southwest France. These are the castles that were built on high peaks and crags by the heretical Cathars in the Middle Ages, and they are steeped in history, drama and mystery. Getting from one to another is a challenging walk over ancient pathways, through lush valleys and over steep hillsides. It is exhilarating, and at times the going gets a little tough, but overall the journey is not too difficult for people like Sally who have a reasonable standard of fitness and can make progress at their own pace. Walkers recuperate each evening with good food and wine in local villages.

Their second trip, in 2007, took them to the north of Spain and eight days of walking the last 100 kilometres of The Camino de Santiago or The Way of St James, which is a magnet to walkers from all over the world who spend days, weeks or months on this historic route.

Next, in 2009, Sally was off to southern Spain to walk among the many little white Moorish villages that dot the countryside of the Andalucia region.

Each of the three trips consisted of about eight days of slow walking, covering 10 to as much as 20 kilometres a day over all sorts of terrain. All three more than exceeded expectations, but nevertheless they threw up challenges that at times taxed the Sally's courage and energy. Bad weather, slippery ground, and the very real possibility of misunderstanding directions and getting lost in remote countryside, were all part of the mix that could have tipped any day into a bad day for the less than intrepid had she not been armed with good advice and great trip notes.

'Sometimes I was exhausted, soaked through with my boots caked in mud, and worrying I wouldn't make it to the next stop, but mostly it was just fantastic. Day after day of fascinating and exhilarating experiences.'

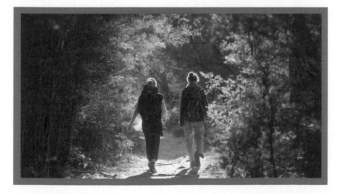

Walkers in the magnificent Freycinet National Park, Tasmania. Photo Freycinet Experience.

Final thoughts ...

If I could not walk far and fast, I think I should just explode and perish.
Charles Dickens

The best remedy for a short temper is a long walk.
Jacqueline Schiff

Methinks that the moment my legs begin to move,
my thoughts begin to flow.
Henry David Thoreau

When I hit a fitness rut, I call a friend to meet me for a walk. It always
helps to make exercising a social opportunity!
Laura Leighton

I have two doctors, my left leg and my right.
G. M. Trevelyan

Walking is good for solving problems –
it's like the feet are little psychiatrists.
Pepper Giardino

My grandmother started walking five miles a day when she was sixty.
She's ninety-three today and we don't know where the hell she is.
Ellen DeGeneres

Index

WONDER WALKERS

In order to encourage people to walk, four-times World Open squash champion Dame Susan Devoy founded Wonder Walkers in 2003 with Paula Thompson. A support and information organisation, Wonder Walkers is the one-stop shop for women and walking, providing both motivational encouragement and practical information for women who want to improve their health and fitness. Experts in physiology, nutrition and other key aspects of health contribute their valuable expertise to the site, which has attracted members from around the world.

Visit the site and join now!

www.wonderwalkers.co.nz

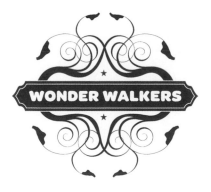

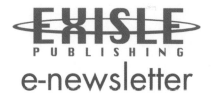

e-newsletter

If you love books as much as we do, why not subscribe to our weekly e-newsletter?

As a subscriber, you'll receive special offers and discounts, be the first to hear of our exciting upcoming titles, and be kept up to date with book tours and author events. You will also receive unique opportunities exclusive to subscribers – and much more!

To subscribe in Australia or from any other country except New Zealand, visit www.exislepublishing.com.au/newsletter-sign-up

For New Zealand, visit
www.exislepublishing.co.nz/newsletter-subscribe